SHRINK

Become Bulletproof,
Move Mountains, and
Create a Revolution Inside Your Body
For The World To See

Daphne Erhart PsyD, M.A.

This book is dedicated to every brave and beautiful soul ready to take the path of true and lasting wellness. I recognize your courage, honesty, and love for yourself and the world and I'm so excited that you are taking this step and starting this journey!

This book is also dedicated to my parents. Your loving dedication to raising a healthy family way before it was the "popular" thing to do has added years to our life and life to our years!

Finally, I am so grateful for my incredibly loving family and friends who have endlessly encouraged and helped me with this project. You are a priceless treasure and you make this world a better place. I am so lucky to have your light in my life. I love you!

About This Book

Are you ready to increase your energy and become healthy and fit like never before? Do you feel a sense of purpose and mission for your life but have not had the energy or health to fully live what you are truly passionate about? If so, this book is for you! This book will get you back in touch with your real inner power and how you make this world a better place. The first step to fulfilling your purpose in life and being fully present for your loved ones is taking charge and taking care of your own life. By changing yourself first, you naturally start to improve the world around you! This world needs you to be fully alive and living your purpose! I'm sure you have seen people who have such amazing abilities, talents, and desires to change the world and make this world a better place but health struggles have kept them from living up to their full potential. Thank you for your bravery and dedication in this first step. The world needs you!

We are in charge of what we do and responsible for most outcomes in our lives. Do you agree? If so, you are going to love the feeling as you read further and realize how powerful you truly are! During this journey, you may process some new or old feelings as we repair the potholes that have slowed you down during past attempts to meet your goals. As you start to realize that you are moving forward towards your clear goals, you may start to feel confident and comfortable with the new you. You may also start to feel very uncomfortable, scared, and possibly doubtful about yourself and the future at times along the journey. Remember that whatever you are feeling is ok. Don't spend too much energy judging or interpreting your feelings. You are not your feelings. Having a roller coaster of feelings is just part of the process of change. Feelings are what they are. They do not rule us. The key is to notice an emotion and let it pass on by without taking ownership as your identity. We experience feelings and yet we are not our feelings.

Continue taking steps towards your goals no matter what emotions come up. Put massive energy into your goal! Stay focused and keep reading through the process while letting your mind soak it in and feel comfortable with the new you. You are always in charge of you no matter what emotional cloud may be floating by at the moment!

Make the choice to join this adventure and the security of knowing that you can have the fit and healthy body you dream of. Take an honest look as you read each chapter, and make the internal decision to change. Learn exactly what you want and why you want it. Then you will have the ammunition you need to do whatever it takes to make the changes you are determined to get! Participate in this journey when you are ready and use this book as a resource and support as you experience real change and live your ideal healthy life.

If what you are reading is uncomfortable or feels confrontational at times, please realize that this may be because at some level you have recognized something within you already that is changing. When you feel this way, you may have already started doing the work needed to make deep, internal changes, and you are already moving in the right direction! You are ready to take advantage of this opportunity as you follow your path to immense health and letting your fit, gorgeous self shine!

Contents

Chapter 1

Create a Revolution Inside your Body for the World to See

You cannot solve a problem from the same consciousness that created it. You must learn to see the world anew. - Albert Einstein

What the mind can conceive and believe, the mind can achieve regardless of how many times you may have failed in the past. -Napoleon Hill

Take the first step in faith. You don't have to see the whole staircase, just take the first step.
-Dr. Martin Luther King Jr.

Have you ever known someone who was born with so many advantages and given so much in life that they could have succeeded with their eyes closed, but were still unsuccessful? Have you ever heard of someone who came from a completely disadvantaged background but defied the odds and became a stunning success? What is the difference between these two people?

Every day more and more exercise programs, diets, self help books, and new health discoveries tell us what new diet, workout, or miracle product will help us have the body of our dreams. Meanwhile, people are becoming more and more unhealthy. How can this be possible? We live in a society where being unhealthy is the norm! If we have so much information and tools available to live a healthy and long life, why is it that instead of improving our condition, we are getting worse?

What if the latest diet, a newly discovered supplement, breaking health news, or the latest workout program is not really what we need? What if the main obstacles to living our ideal lives is really inside ourselves?

Are these thoughts scary to you, or does it make you feel excited and powerful? Let me tell you a secret. If most of what we need to change is inside of us, we are in luck! If the change we need is already inside ourselves, we are truly able to start making changes now. It is totally within our control.

Most people are attracted to fitness programs because they want to lose weight to look good. Although it is always nice to feel good about the way you look, there are so many more powerful reasons to stick with a healthy lifestyle.

The goal of this book is to help you reclaim your power. The goal is to prevent this oozing problem from getting bigger, not by putting a band-aid on it, but by curing it at its source. This book will get to the bottom of this downward spiral and start getting the momentum moving in the right direction!

Multiple Personality Disorder or Dissociative Identity Disorder is a fascinating (and very rare) phenomenon. It is a psychological phenomenon where people develop separate personalities within themselves, usually in response to experiencing deep trauma. One of the most fascinating aspects of multiple personalities is that even the person's physical characteristics can change! It is a prime example of the link between the mind and body.

As a person switches from one personality to another, new physiological patterns have been measured to change as quickly as the person changes from one personality to another. This includes their heart rate, breath rate, physical ticks, physical idiosyncrasies, posture, strength, handwriting, and allergies. These physiological changes can happen within a couple of minutes. Imagine now what physical changes you can make within a day, a week, a year from doing the internal work and changing from the inside out!

The lasting change we need is internal instead of external. Once thinking and feeling in healthy ways becomes an ingrained part of our personality, it naturally becomes our lifestyle. Imagine if you were able to make something click inside so that you genuinely want and crave the very things that make you healthy! Once the mind and heart changes and no more flimsy band-aids are used to fix or cure an internal problem, the changes will flow naturally. Start to let your mind wander to what a fit person would think, feel, and do from day to day. Then your actions will flow out naturally to support you and match your inner fitness!

Let me tell you another secret. Successful people develop a personalized approach to fitness. In other words, a "one-size-fits-all" recommendation of any type (diet, supplement, bootcamp, etc.) rarely works long term unless it is personalized, enjoyable, and part of a long term lifestyle. Follow the basic steps in this book and workbook that will help you develop a personalized long term lifestyle that you research, create, and enjoy for the rest of your life.

Make sure you filter all suggestions from other people on how to change your life before you decide to take them in. Fitting into someone else's mold and conforming your body, mind, and spirit to another human's desire can be disrespectful to yourself.   Decide whether or not their thoughts, values, or suggestions are something you agree with before you commit to digest and fully processing it. Deep down you know what is best for you more than anyone else. Respect your body. Respect your heart. Respect yourself. You deserve it.

No matter what physical condition you believe your body is in right now, it is important to show yourself some love NOW. Our body's health depends not only on what we feed it and how we move it, but how we think and feel about it!

Respect and thank your body for always being there for you. Your body is a phenomenal machine. If you are alive and reading this, you have so much to thank your body for! There is immense beauty and strength already in you right now to recognize. Do not wait until you meet an outside standard to love and respect yourself. You are already gorgeous just the way you are.

Begin this new lifestyle from a point of abundance, not with feelings of lack or desperation. Start to be in charge of your own emotions and views of yourself today. Work out this muscle of appreciating your body now, and you will start an upward spiral of success.

Be your own best advocate and champion. Be careful not to swallow what the media and cultural ideals feed you without first processing what is going into your unconscious mind. Your thoughts and feelings are immensely powerful.

Decide to love and respect yourself and your body no matter what. Look at yourself in the mirror. Look at your amazing skin. Embrace your entire body. Feel the breath of life flow in and out of your lungs. Notice your own emotion and passion shining out of your eyes.

Acknowledge what your phenomenal body does for you every second of every day. Notice how your brain can quickly process new concepts and new ways of being. Recognize that your heart and emotions are in sync and important part of your intuition. Look deep into your own eyes in the mirror and recognize the greatness within you.

In this sometimes crazy, unpredictable world, the process of becoming healthy is different than what we are used to. We are used to learning the answers from other "experts". We are used to people who have studied something for years telling us how to live and what to believe. That is the first mistake. Yes, there are some basic scientific facts that can be useful, but living a healthy lifestyle is actually an internal revolution that is totally in our own control.

Although our environment influences us, the good news is that you have the final say with your own body. Your health is not based on the economy, how anyone feels about you, your job, or anything else. You get all the credit now when you make this internal change and begin this adventure!

Deep down, we know what we need to do to live a truly vibrant, energetic, gorgeously healthy lifestyle. **What we need is a revolution deep inside that shifts our deepest ways of being and existing, so that our natural blueprint is to be healthy, happy, and living in our dream body.** This internal change is a fresh, permanent, new way of living. This internal revolution involves permanently adopting some of the things that make us truly feel good into our everyday lives and feeling deeply happy and satisfied from day to day! Remember-it's not about what you know, it's how you internalize and use it!

If you are wanting to be sold on the latest diet, workout program, or supplement, this is not the book for you. This journey will be in your control and you can succeed if you truly want to. Most everyone knows the basic concepts of eating healthfully and calories in vs. calories out. The problem isn't usually about not **knowing** the actions and principles of weight loss to become our ideal, healthy self. The solution is addressing what it is that truly keeps our actions from matching our knowledge about what we need to do.

If you do not feel ready to make an internal change at this time, are on the fence about it, or want to learn about weight loss intellectually without making any real internal or external change, this book is not for you. If you really want a miracle pill and would like to continue trying one after the other, please move on. If you are content being overweight, underweight, tired, or cutting down the years you have yet to live your life, please don't read any further.

However, if you truly want emotional and mental change and you want to live a different, full, colorful, congruent, blissful and vibrant life, read on! You don't need all the answers before you start. Just continue reading with an open heart. You will take your own personalized steps as you read and finish this book. You will be surprised at how things naturally change as you read each chapter and develop your personalized fitness plan.

As a psychologist, I've been told repeatedly not to go into the fitness and weight loss field because due to the physical nature of the human body, it takes the longest time to see results. Please realize that even when you have already made a real and permanent internal change to support a new body, you don't see results immediately. It simply takes some time to lose or gain weight due to basic biology. Keep up the good work and remember that gorgeous results will be visible soon. The results can be permanent when you have patience with yourself and stay strong and motivated regardless of immediate rewards!

In other words, once someone has made the internal, permanent change and becomes a "fit" person on the inside, it usually takes months to see the final result of their body matching their inner self. A human body can shed or gain weight only so fast. You are not going to lose or gain 30 pounds overnight even if you have completely changed your lifestyle and internal blueprint. However, when you have made the internal change and kept it long term so that you do see results, it is immensely rewarding!

This means that when you are living your new self congruently from the inside out, your outside body will definitely reflect the inside if you keep at it and give yourself time for your new body to develop.

It may have taken you months, years, or your entire life to create the body you have currently, so even when you immediately start realizing and living your ideal self, it may take a little while to see the ultimate end result you imagine (depending on how far from your ideal self you start out at). Keep in your mind what you are working towards at all times. Do not indulge yourself in thinking about what you are moving away from. Focusing on your goal will catapult you towards it. You will start living what you are letting into your mind and heart every day.

Inside Change = Outside Change. Neither inside change or outside change are available in pill form! Up until now, you may not have been living your ideal life in your ideal body. Your ideal self still exists inside of you. If you are ready to let your ideal self rule your life now, read on to begin this massive and exciting internal shift. Enjoy the ride as you begin to see, feel, and know deep down that you are a fit and gorgeous person every day of your life.

You may have heard that our thoughts produce our emotions. You may have also heard the opposite--that our emotions impact what we think about or experience. What do you think? Which one is most important--our emotions or our thoughts? It is like the question of which one came first--the chicken or the egg? Is it the thought or the feeling that comes first? Both our thoughts and feelings influence each other. Our thoughts and emotions not only have a great impact on our body, but taking initial steps such as exercise and eating well affects our mind and body. Get the most bang for your buck by not only taking action when you don't feel like it but also changing your mindset and getting into the habit of experiencing positive emotions that motive positive actions regardless of your circumstances. Tackling this from both directions will give you the most progress.

Do you ever notice that the day after you have treated your body badly, you may feel less motivated, have more negative mood swings, and/or have less mental clarity? It's not all in your head! Treating your body well will help you in other aspects of your life such as thinking clearly or making good decisions rapidly, which will give you an edge to stay on track. A friend of mine, a winner of several worldwide fitness competitions, wakes himself up each morning at 5:30am to exercise and lift weights for an hour and eat a healthy breakfast before he begins work. He says it is the one thing that guarantees that he will have a good day.

Another friend of mine does not work out unless he feels like it. He does not disturb his sleep in the morning. Since he has created an overall healthy lifestyle, his body now naturally craves movement and substantial foods that provide nutrients throughout the day. He ends up working out later in the day several times a week and eating healthfully by being in tune with and listening to what his body wants.

Which one does it correctly? Both! They have both found what works best for them. If there were negative results, then it might be a good idea to tweak it so that they can get the results they are looking for. They are both getting the desired outcome by doing different things. There is no right or wrong answer to this. You are the judge of your own body and life and you get to make the decisions. If you are really honest with yourself in this journey and can realize that experimenting (trial and error) can take you in the right direction, you will start to detect most quickly what is best for you.

Sometimes you may detect a feeling that will make you want to change your behavior. Other times, you may notice that a certain habit you create starts to make you feel even more motivated and happy! What you do and what you feel is intertwined and influence each other.

To summarize, don't wait to feel a certain way before you take action AND don't take action at the expense of ignoring what your body and spirit really need. There is usually a multidirectional interaction between your motivation, feelings, and actions. Actions and feelings are not usually one simple cause=effect situation.

For example, exercise and eating right will likely improve your mood. In turn, your improved mood can help you stay motivated by strengthening your mind and emotions so that you will form a positive spiral and want to continue your new way of eating and exercising in the long run.

Listening to what makes you feel best is the smart way to go. Instead of forcing your body, heart, and brain to conform to a process that fits into someone else's box, feed it what it needs and wants. Respecting yourself in this way results in wanting to do it more often, which keeps on improving your health! Repeating things that improve your mood and mindset also help keep you on track for the long haul.

Chapter 2

Move Mountains

Champions aren't made in gyms. Champions are made from something they have deep inside them--a desire, a dream, a vision. They have to have the skill, and the will. But the will must be stronger than the skill.
-Muhammad Ali

How wonderful it is that nobody need wait a single moment before starting to improve the world. -Anne Frank

The world as we have created it is a process of our thinking. It cannot be changed without changing our thinking. -Albert Einstein

Have you ever decided to try something completely new and been successful at it? I'm sure you can think of something--driving a car, earning a degree, becoming a parent, learning how to walk for the first time? There is always that initial learning curve where you see a glimpse of how you will have to learn or change something to be successful. You may not be an expert on the first try, but you know that you have what you need to learn, make that internal shift, and become good at it with some practice.

Your ability to try something completely new and succeed is a skill you already have. You are now going to expand to your way of thinking, feeling, and being regarding your physical body and eventually be successful with your health. When you were a baby learning to walk, you first had to learn to crawl, stand, and then taking steps and fall. Falling and tripping once in a while learning to walk was just part of the process of getting to your goal of walking.

During this process of creating a new internal health blueprint, going slowly at times, and "failing" other times are all just a part of the process of learning how to be very good at taking care of your body! Setbacks are actually signs you are going in the right direction and will be successful.

You can move mountains. You can create a revolution inside your body that changes your physical body. You can let your body release weight it doesn't need and gain muscle that is good for your body. You can create days full of energy and vibrance. All you need is to believe it, have a strong enough reason to do it, and never stop taking action!

What is your personal reason to become more healthy? Everyone's way of becoming motivated is different. Take a few minutes right now and think about how you expect your life to be once you are living in your ideal body.

Some reasons may include:

"I want to have enough energy to meet my goals!"

"I want to live an active life until I'm at least 100 years old!"

"I want to enjoy the lifestyle I had ten years ago"

"Hiking Mount Kilimanjaro is on my bucket list"

"I want to feel self confident moving and living in my own body"

"I want to be physically able to play and do things with my children outdoors!"

"I want to defeat my family tendency to get diabetes [or any other hereditary health condition] and I know that losing weight will help."

"I want my body to be able to keep up with my mind when I'm working"

"I've tried to lose weight and relapsed in the past, so I want to prove to myself that I can actually change my lifestyle for good!"

"I want to feel free--no longer be trapped inside the limitations of my body"

"I want to have more energy and feel more alive"

"I want to feel more attractive and sexy!"

Success has to do more with the "why" you pursue it than the "how". There are usually many ways to meet a health goal. Only the dedicated will do what it takes to keep going until they find the right path for them to meet their particular goal. As Mohammad Ali stated, the "will" must be greater than the "skill". In other words, wake up and listen to that powerful voice inside you and become your own superman or wonder woman whenever you want to! Your incredible motivation will produce a power that surpasses anything that intellectualizing, philosophizing, or following someone else's personal recipe for success could ever bring. In order to succeed, your reason WHY needs to be that strong number one desire for your life.

Have you ever been in a situation where your inner super man or wonder woman woke up and you made the impossible happen? Did you notice someone in danger or an injustice and felt you just HAD to take action and couldn't keep walking by? A person can do almost anything if their reason is strong enough. For example, if you truly believe it is a matter of life and death, your reason to change your life immediately becomes strong enough to move mountains, not to mention change your eating habits!

It is important to educate yourself to find out what is really good for you in any aspect in your life. For example, you could read about the Paleo diet, becoming vegan or vegetarian, learn about HIIT workouts, benefits of sleep, water, whole organic foods, etc. However, the main reasons for failure is usually not related to not knowing enough.

People who have access to infinite information fail because they have not taken

strong enough, lasting action. In order to stay on track for the rest of your life, your new lifestyle needs to fully support your new primary goal. It is a systemic life makeover!

When you stay focused on why you want to move toward your goal, it will create a lifestyle that will give you exactly what you want. Not only do you need that initial realization and clear motivation of why you are doing this, you need to keep this in the front of your mind day in and day out. Keep reminders on your bathroom mirror, refrigerator, or cell phone. **Tell loved ones and supportive people in your life the REASON for your health goals so that they can remind you later.**

Let people you trust hold you accountable and always remember that you must always be doing this foremost for yourself. It may also affect your loved ones in a positive way when you are energetic, physically fit, and feeling good about yourself. However, your personal reasons and desires for yourself are most effective when they are the main things that drive you.

My father was diagnosed with multiple myeloma, a particular type of cancer that is systemic throughout the bone marrow of his entire body.

"Experts" said that this cancer never goes into "remission". Before his diagnosis, he would enjoy pizza and junk food on occasion, and poke fun of people who were too particular about what they ate.

Although he was fairly healthy before the cancer diagnosis, he made a DRASTIC and complete change in his eating habits immediately after being diagnosed. He was in the hospital in a very serious condition and according to statistics, the prognosis was poor even after being provided a bone marrow transplant and other medical treatment. As you can imagine, he felt awful physically and in addition, learning that he had cancer was emotionally devastating.

He knew that he needed to make serious lifestyle changes and that this was a matter of life and death due to the systemic type of cancer that he had. He decided wholeheartedly to make whatever drastic changes were needed in his lifestyle. Even though he was feeling badly, he immediately put his mind to doing research and quickly learned about the relation of diet and exercise to cancer. From that moment forward, he ate only pure, nutritious foods, without exception. He drank alkaline water, did not eat animal products (not even dairy due to how it promotes inflammation) and COMPLETELY cut out sugar and artificial sweeteners of any kind from his diet.

After eight months since he had last eaten pizza or even a bite of a candy bar, he told me this story about what he went through earlier that week in the grocery store parking lot. At that point, my dad felt he had "survived". His cancer was still there but not as strong as before. He was relieved that his health had made significant improvement.

In a moment of weakness at the grocery store, he picked up his favorite delicious chocolate candy bar as he waited in line to check out. He reasoned to himself, "I haven't eaten a candy bar in more than 8 months and I deserve to have one after all I've been through, especially now that the cancer is not as strong and my body has regained strength. In the big scheme of things, what could one candy bar do to my body anyway?" He sat in the car slowly unwrapping the tasty chocolate bar. He was so excited to finally taste it again after so long. As he unwrapped it, his mouth started watering. He started smelling some of the melted chocolate on his fingers.

In that moment, he realized that he could easily eat the candy bar if he wanted to. There was nothing and nobody that could stop him. He could throw the wrapper in the trash can a few feet away and nobody would even know that he had eaten it. At that moment, he also started remembering what he had learned about sugar – that it creates an acidic environment in the body that cancer thrives on. He imagined the cancer cells in his body being so happy that they were about to get sugar so that the cancer cells could become big and strong again. He imagined the little cancer cells excitedly cheering, "Yay! We are finally getting sugar so we can survive and grow big and strong again. I can't wait!"

That visualization was the turning point for my Dad! As much as he wanted to eat the delicious candy bar, his motivation to continue to live became so strong that he could no longer eat the candy bar. He truly wanted to live more than anything else, especially more than a momentary indulgence of the chocolate.

My dad's desire to live was so strong and congruent that all other cravings, feelings, and reasoning could not keep him from staying away from sugar, which he wholeheartedly believed would give the cancer cells the ability to thrive again in his body. If you truly believed you were in a life or death situation, could you stay away from sugar for 8 minutes? 8 months? 8 years?

It is humanly possible to do anything as long as there is a strong enough reason to do it. By the way, almost 12 years later (at the time this book is published), he has outlived most people who were diagnosed with multiple myeloma around the same time as him. His recent tests now reveal a more healthy body chemistry, probably due to his commitment to clean eating and walking three miles outdoors every day no matter how he felt.

We can do just about anything if we put our mind to it and if we believe in it wholeheartedly. Our reasons to do something are much more powerful than any excuses.

Let me tell you about a tough time in my life when I was feeling sorry for myself. I was in the process of divorce. I was heartbroken, stressed, and felt a huge lack of meaningful emotional support that I desperately needed during that time. I still had about six months of my full time psychology internship to complete before finally getting my doctorate degree. The stakes were high. If I didn't successfully complete this internship, I would not get the degree that I had been working on for the last 7 years, yet I would still have about $200,000 in student loan debt I would have to somehow repay for the rest of my life. I would never be able to live that beautiful dream of being a psychologist if I didn't successfully finish this demanding internship. It was crunch time in my life. I was almost there and I HAD to finish.

To make ends meet and have a place to live, I lived and worked at a retirement facility dealing with medical emergencies during the night while also working full daytime hours completing my psychology internship, helping people with major psychological problems meet their personal goals every weekday. I had just turned 30 years old and was always physically and emotionally EXHAUSTED!

Early one morning before the sun came up, I was delivering newspapers to the residents before leaving for my internship. I slowly and sleepily walked through the hallway dropping a newspaper at every door wishing I had the time to sleep, work out at the gym, and do more things to take care of my physical self, not to mention my emotional depletion. I was heartbroken, lonely, and exhausted. I had excuses in my head.

It was a quiet, early morning, and I started to hear shuffling coming from behind me. I was walking as fast as I could delivering the papers so I could finish and get to my internship on time but someone was walking fast and gaining on me from behind. This was very rare at that retirement facility. I was usually the one who moved the fastest.

As I sleepily kept putting one foot in front of the other, a resident whom I knew was 105 years old passed me, giving me a cheerful "Good morning"! She was doing her morning walk down the halls of our building and with the help of her walker, she passed me!

That was a huge wakeup call for me. I quickly laughed at myself inside and reminded myself that **"there are no excuses". When you put your mind to something, you just do it!**

Sure, I may have been dealing with immense stress, but there was living proof that someone 75 years older than me and over the age of 100 certainly didn't feel sorry for herself or give herself any excuses. She always had a positive attitude and had recently been featured in the National Geographic magazine pumping her own gas into her car. What did I have to complain about? A little morning walk that ultimately made me exercise, which reduces stress? Little did she know that her morning walk and cheerful greeting helped change my mindset that morning. She was living proof that anything is possible when you decide it is.

What mountain do you decide to move today? And more importantly, WHY? What is the reason that will keep you motivated in years to come?

Chapter 3

Does it give you goosebumps?

If you don't know where you're going, any road'll take you there. -George Harrison

You gain strength, courage, and confidence by every experience in which you really stop to look fear in the face. You must do the things which you think you cannot do.
-Eleonor Roosevelt

Some people dream of success, while others wake up and work hard at it! -Winston Churchill

Do you get a wave of excitement, a huge smile spreading across your face, and goosebumps when you think of what your body will be like in a few weeks or months from now?

Have you heard the story of Major Nesmith? He was a prisoner of war in Vietnam held in solitary confinement for 7 years. During those long years, to keep himself sane, he imagined himself playing a round of golf every day. He would imagine playing 18 holes of golf in great detail. He would start by imagining himself going to his closet to get his golf clubs, and then imagine in detail every single step he would take to get to the golf course, every breath, where he would look, the direction of the wind, color of the grass, the particular angle he would swing, and how he would follow through and make his shot. He did this in detail for about 5 hours a day. After 7 years, he was finally released back home.

Even though he had not actually played golf in over 7 years, he had visualized himself playing in his mind. When he played for the first time after returning home, he had actually significantly improved his game!

His friends were absolutely shocked when he played his first game after returning. He should have been a lot worse since he was out of practice and had just gone through an incredibly stressful ordeal for years.

When you really think about it, excellent athletes begin their winning games inside. Although Major Nesmith could not physically practice for years, he had years and years of expert experience visualizing perfect games in his mind. This goes to show how important our internal game is. Visualizing in detail what our desired outcome will be is extremely powerful in physically transforming our body and meeting goals!

Create a picture in your mind of what you will look like once you have met your amazing fitness goal. How might everyday activities feel differently? What emotions will you feel when you look in the mirror? How might people see and relate to you? What styles and colors of clothes are you wearing when you visualize your future self? What will it feel like when your body has more muscle and less fat and you are able to do things and move in ways you weren't able to before?

Make your "What" strong enough to get you out of bed every morning. A strong "what" is always focused on the positive and can give you goosebumps when you let yourself really dwell on the possibilities!

Concentrate and become clear on what exactly your goal is and what habits you will develop to achieve and keep that goal long term. Always focus on how to do things right rather than what you want to avoid. You will automatically gravitate towards what you think about so make sure you are always visualizing what you actually want in your life!

Have you ever watched a great athlete who only thinks about all of the mistakes he or she could possibly make before every competition or game? Of course not! The good athletes and champions have developed an excellent skill in visualizing exactly what they want even before they take physical action. They have already created the success in their mind and lead their body to replicate what they have already envisioned for themselves.

Let's imitate these athletes! They know that to be successful, they need to visualize in the positive, and not the negative. In your own success journey, create and clearly visualize a physical goal that really makes you extremely excited, focused, and motivated.

It is imperative that you have a clear vision of what you want to become. Can you become something that you cannot even imagine? How can one meet a goal that hasn't even been created? Meeting a goal is done by taking action, and actions come from thoughts. Thoughts come from beliefs and attitudes. Make your goals amazing, awe-inspiring, and the number one thing that you live for and get out of bed for every morning.

A positive goal with strong emotion can give you boundless energy and power. Think about it--if you are your own worst critic all day every day, making yourself aware of every bad thing about you, not wanting to look into the mirror, and feeling more and more horrible about yourself as the day goes on, your energy will wither away and become consumed by that negativity you have generated. However, having a clear picture of what you want will give you immense excitement, energy, and anticipation.

If you are trying to feel better but are concentrating on the negativity, after a while, you will become tired, maybe sick, and will need a break from it all. Doing things while feeling negative and avoidant makes you weaker, while appreciating any good and beautiful qualities about yourself and building on that feeling more and more makes you stronger. There is always something to appreciate and build on about yourself!

Right now, stop for a moment and notice every good thing about yourself that you can think of for one minute. Include both internal (e.g. integrity, love, and other qualities of character) and external qualities (e.g. eyes, skin,

movement, hair, smile, frame, muscles, etc.).
Enjoy how magnificent you are for a few
moments.

Have you heard of the little girl once named
Norma Jean? She lived in orphanages and
foster care. She didn't have many nice things,
and is quoted as saying, "no-one ever told me I
was pretty when I was a little girl. All little girls
should be told they're pretty, even if they aren't".
She was just a little girl from the country whose
mother was in an insane asylum. She never
knew her father. There are millions of girls in the
world from all walks of life who dream of
becoming a or beauty icon. How did this little girl
become the timeless beauty icon, Marilyn
Monroe?

First of all, she knew exactly what she wanted.
She had a dream. She didn't become an icon
because she was traditionally more beautiful
than any other girl. She became who we now
know as Marilyn Monroe because of what was
going on inside of her. She lived and breathed
her dream every single day. Her mannerisms,
her new name, her way of speaking and relating
to people, and her choice of clothes and
hairstyle, and her career choices all came from
the strong vision she had since childhood and

her commitment to act and be who she was meant to be. She eventually embodied what she focused on every second of her life. It made her excited and motivated every time she thought about it as a little girl. Norma Jean didn't let anyone sidetrack her until she became Marilyn Monroe.

As human, we nurture ourselves in many ways, one of which is food. This can be healthy or unhealthy depending on what your mind, body, and spirit really need! When you start to crave or want food, start to become aware of how your body is feeling. Also, make a habit of becoming aware of your emotions and what your spirit is longing for in that moment. It could be that your body needs a number of things but isn't aware of exactly what it truly needs. Some overlooked needs are undisturbed sleep, sex, emotional connection, a sense of belonging or connection, a sense of value and contributing to this world, or simply physical exertion to get rid of stress. You may really need to cry, scream, laugh, hug, have sex, be held, or be told you are loved and amazing. You may need to feel acknowledged and respected for everything you did that day or in your lifetime to become who you are. You may need something to look forward to, more excitement, or a more significant life purpose so that you feel alive and know you are contributing something great to the world. Start to pay attention to what you really need. Listen to yourself and nurture your true desires and needs. Become an expert at identifying what you really want and need and then fulfill that by nurturing yourself in many ways in addition to food. These ways can range from physical to emotional to interpersonal. For example, getting a massage, a bath, yoga, sleep, aromatherapy, lotions, freshly squeezed juices, a comfortable office chair, a cozy blanket, a walk in the sun, choosing to only spend significant time with people who treat others with respect and genuine care, forgiving yourself for mistakes, celebrating a success, saying loving and encouraging things to yourself, or cuddling with a pet.

Becoming good at identifying and fulfilling your true needs and wants is key to living a healthy lifestyle for the rest of your life. If you do not develop ways other than food or drink to feel satisfied and nurtured and truly content, you may be setting yourself up for failure. Treat yourself with kindness and respect at all times. Because if you don't, you will need even more nurturing at the end of the day. Beating yourself up internally all day makes it harder (not easier) to resist cravings.

I know some people who restrict themselves ruthlessly. They would not even dare treat a child the same way they treat themselves. They may drastically cut back on calories, say critical things to themselves as they see their reflection in a window or mirror, berate themselves with every movement that reminds them of what they want to change in their body, and then expect themselves to wake up feeling bright and cheerful the next day. The next day of this type of cycle gets worse if not corrected, beating themselves up again and making a stronger resolution for more self-deprivation to avoid feeling so badly again.

This can't go on forever! The body needs some nurturing for survival (not to mention nourishment) and the inevitable "binge" contributes to more negative feelings and a resolution to eat even less (when in fact it most likely isn't a true "binge"--just the body's desire to nurture and sustain itself). You are human and you do need food. Just learn to do it in ways that make you feel energized, satisfied, and feel wonderful about yourself. In future chapters you will begin to outline the type of lifestyle you can create that will give you results you need.

It is important to love yourself no matter what stage you are in this process. Unconditional love for your own self will give you the energy and internal strength you need to get through anything. Forgive yourself for not being perfect and for anything that you have in your memory that you have ever done wrong. We cannot do anything about the past.

Ho'oponopono is a Hawaiian process of forgiveness. Give yourself some quiet time undisturbed by anyone else, look into your own eyes in a mirror and repeat this simple, yet powerful process of Ho'oponopono. Look at yourself as a loving parent would look at their precious child. Repeat these words several times. Repeat the words slowly and with meaning while looking into your own eyes:

I'm sorry.
Please forgive me.
Thank you.
I love you.

Simple, yet powerfully healing. Forgiveness does not mean that what was done is ok. It simply means you are releasing it and that you will move on to make the rest of your life as

much of a blessing to you and those around you
as possible.

Starting today, spend at least 15 minutes in the
morning and 15 minutes in the evening every day
by yourself in a comfortable, pleasant place
where you feel safe and nurtured. During these
15 minutes, visualize your ideal healthy, fit body.
Let yourself fully experience how it feels to move
and live in your ideal body. Visualize in detail
what you look like, how you interact with others,
what you think to yourself when you look into the
mirror, and how good you now feel about
yourself. Start to notice how good you feel.
Notice that spark of joy, love, internal motivation,
and appreciation for yourself radiating from your
chest throughout your entire body. Notice how it
makes you feel deeply content and happy with
who you are right now. Do this every day starting
now.

Chapter 4

The Good News Is - It's All Your Fault!

We are what we pretend to be, so we must be careful about what we pretend to be.
-Kurt Vonnegut

Better to get hurt by the truth than comforted with a lie. -Khaled Hosseini

In the end, we shape our lives, and we shape ourselves. The process never ends until we die. And the choices we make are ultimately our own responsibility. -Eleanor Roosevelt

How would it feel to know that everything that exists in your life is entirely your fault? First of all, relax. It is time to realize that there are certain things you have experienced that you could not control, the most obvious being habits formed as a baby and child. Both good and bad habits are often formed very early in life. Some are lucky enough to have had parents who help them form great habits and others not so much.

Eating habits are one of the most automatic, ingrained things that we learn starting at birth (before birth, technically). Patterns of eating are started even before you can remember! They are very automatic and powerful, and by adulthood, they have often become complex and automatic. There are so many interactions of variables that lead to the development of what goes on inside us. Some of which are our emotions, thoughts, physical feelings and cravings. The inner blueprint of how we interact with food, exercise, and other factors that influence metabolism can be different from person to person.

Habits formed in childhood range from patterns of eating, drinking, sleeping, and physical activity. They are linked to connecting with others, coping with stress, boredom, pleasure, the basic instinct of comforting oneself, and dealing with traumas or repeated discomfort. Food is a very basic source of comfort. Eating is usually one of the first ways a baby experiences being comforted, loved, and connected to their caregiver.

Also, keep in mind that everyone deals with experiences differently in life. For example, someone who has been severely deprived in the past, may have an unconscious desire to "hoard" or gather as much as possible since they do not know when the next available source of nourishment will be. Since food can be linked to many emotional and interpersonal needs, some which were listed above, it may have become a substitute for something else that was lacking.

Another example is how food is sometimes used to manage difficult emotions. Sometimes feeling unable to express emotions such as anger or neediness can result in "stuffing" the feelings by using food. This can happen particularly if there is any type of physical, sexual, emotional, or mental abuse. Also, being deprived of a supportive atmosphere to express genuine thoughts and feelings and be supported when we need it the most can trigger other ways of coping, often including using food.

One thing that keeps some people overweight without them fully realizing it is fear of being strongly desired physically and sexually. The excess weight may unconsciously be used as a form of protection for whatever reason (sometimes past or anticipated abuse or trauma). This may be the case especially if you have experienced trauma as a child or adult. The good news is that now things are different! You are no longer helpless.

If you are an adult reading this, you now have the choice of whether or not to allow people close to you. If you are not an adult yet and have had a traumatic experience like this, please contact a safe person immediately. Depending on the situation, this may mean calling the police, telling a trusted teacher or family member. If you are an adult who has experienced trauma, you may need more support in healing and becoming empowered again. Please do whatever it takes to get the help you need if this is something that you are currently struggling with. You are valuable and worthy of love and respect at all times.

Assuming you are not experiencing trauma any longer, you are now immensely powerful and safe. Now you can experience feeling safe and powerful, which leads to having power to create your life in every way (including your body and health).

Your life is your own! From now on, take responsibility for the good and bad. Forgive your past self and congratulate and celebrate yourself for all you have survived and for the new path that you have taken! When you find one path isn't leading you in the right direction, change your path! Never give up. Try again! It works!

Meeting your goals and making "mistakes" during the process is natural. Think of it like steering a car. Driving and steering is a constant action. You are always turning slightly, correcting the direction to steer you the right way as the road slightly curves or wind blows from different angles. What would happen if you got into the car, measured the exact direction you need to go, pointed the steering wheel precisely in that direction, and never moved it afterwards? You would likely run into a ditch shortly after you begin your journey! Making small and constant "corrections" and movements is what one calls successful driving.

The same goes with life and meeting fitness goals! On day one, you may have it all mapped out and decide how you want the rest of your life to be. Great! On day two, you may realize that it is better to make a small correction in what you eat for lunch in order to give you enough energy so that you are not famished by dinner. Or you may realize that you are not a morning person and need to squeeze in a workout in the middle of the day or go to sleep earlier. Who cares if you "fail" one day. There is no such thing as failure! Failure doesn't exist. It is all just feedback. It just means that you have more information for the next day to learn how to be even more successful! Be open to feedback from yourself so that you will become even better and better.

NOW... the real key is to take initiative inside yourself and focus all of your thoughts and energy not on how you have done things in the past, but on fully taking charge of your life immediately to create the life and fit body you desire and to keep it for the rest of your life.

Don't worry! Being "stuck" in the past was not your fault, but now the key is to realize that **now you can be the source** of everything: action, inaction, and consciously forming habits you choose (not ones that you have been programmed with). It all comes from a deep and complete internal change and there IS something you can do about it. In fact, you have already started!

I'm often asked why people yoyo diet, or to understand why they do such negative things that get them off track. Listen! If you truly want a change, focus on what you want. Don't spend your energy coming up with theories of why you have failed in the past. Of course, it feels good to understand ourselves and why we do what we do, but every person's experience is different and there is not one blanket explanation or theory that would fit for everyone's reason for yoyo dieting, binge eating, or any other problem.

There are many theories out there and the truth is that each person's failure and success is individual and personalized. The best way to reach success is not to find an overarching theory of why things go right or wrong, but to learn and take immediate action and modify things as needed for your particular needs and circumstances.

You are the expert of your own body. Listen to yourself and your true needs and you will start to fulfill them and learn how to take care of yourself and your body properly. Throw your "story" about why you previously failed out the window. Remember that only feedback exists--not failure. Learn what works for you and always MOVE ON!

Here are some reasons for why I won't go into depth on why we do what we do but rather focus on how we can meet our goals.

First of all, there are many reasons for yoyo dieting, binge eating, overeating, etc. These reasons are influenced by a particular person's complex background, personality structure, and inner workings.

Our brains and bodies are very complex, and there is not a one size fits all explanation. There are many aspects that can be involved, such as blood sugar imbalances, emotional overeating, etc. The quick answer is: there is usually an interaction of many reasons AND the reasons depend on the person!

Second of all, deep down, people often know a lot about WHY they yoyo diet or have negative health habits. Wouldn't it be better to be successful at creating and living the lifestyle you want, and understand how you are doing things right so that you can continue this process for the rest of your life?

Most importantly, what we focus on attracts more of the same thing. Ask an addict to talk about how a craving feels or ask them about things they are trying to stay away from and their mind will start to think of and crave that very thing! As a kid, my dad used to jokingly tell me to "think of anything but a white polar bear". A white polar bear was the only thing I could think of! Focus on what you want, rather than what you don't want!

From now on, practice taking responsibility for everything in your life--the good and bad! No more venting about how your ex messed up your life or how things would have been different if you had grown up with a healthier emotional or physical environment. If you are reading this, you have already survived and have taken steps so you can soon be thriving! Take responsibility for where you are today. Realize that what you have learned from your ex or anyone who has done you wrong is invaluable. There is no-one else who has learned that heart lesson quite like you have.

If you have grown up with an extra obstacle, it has only made you stronger and able to know what it really takes to be successful in any circumstance unlike those who have not seen hard times yet. Recognize just how powerful your mind is and the power of a reframe (shifting the way you look at things). What you now believe is your greatest weakness may in fact be your greatest strength in the long run.

Practicing taking responsibility for everything in your life gives you more power. Let yourself live! If your heart gets broken, congratulate yourself and be thankful that you let yourself fully be open to love. If people let you down, be glad that you once were able to be strong enough to trust them. Continue believing in yourself and your ability to learn from mistakes, heal, grow, and love. You are the cause of your body's health at this current moment. Taking responsibility is key to success. From this moment forward, realize that you are powerful beyond measure. From now on, do everything with purpose and a full heart!

Chapter 5

Devour your Cocoon!

When I let go of what I am, I become what I might be. -Lao Tzu

The intuitive mind is a sacred gift and the rational mind a faithful servant. We have created a society that honors the servant and has forgotten the gift -Albert Einstein

New beginnings are often disguised as painful endings. -Lao Tzu

If you are like most people, you have been sleeping in your cocoon for too long! You have nurtured yourself in your cocoon and researched many different ways to change. You know the right things to do to become more healthy and lose weight, and you have educated opinions about the different options, diets, supplements, and types of new exercises regimens! The problem isn't not knowing or studying or researching the right thing to do. It is now time for action. Now is the time to take that first step out of your cocoon and spread your wings!

Think about it--if you want your physical body to be different, you need to take actions and steps you have not yet taken or completed yet. It is time to step out of your comfort zone, shake up your routine, and do what you haven't done before. The key is to DO. It is time to get rid of your cocoon that has been wrapped around you for so long nurturing and protecting you. This step is not something you need more understanding to do.

Take this opportunity to do something new despite fear and uncertainty. Accept the feelings of uncertainty and fear and take action anyway. Moving forward and letting yourself fully experience fear do not have to be mutually exclusive! The worst thing you could do is to wait until those feelings are no longer there to take action.

When will you know that NOW is the time to break out of your comfortable cocoon? How will you know that NOW is the time to make the inner change that you had been waiting for--to change your health and fitness? What you can't do is not to be able to realize this. You should consider that you can do this when you are ready. Can you not?

You are the expert of your own body! Never let anyone else tell you what is best for you. Know yourself. Learn from those who encourage you to become an even better expert on what is right for you and empower you to become healthier and stronger on your own.

Another step you make as you break out of your cocoon is to reframe the definition of failure. "Failure" is simply being one step closer to finding what is right for you! If you try something and it doesn't produce the results you had hoped for, you are much better off than if you had never tried at all because you now can rule that out and move on to what will get you closer to your goal!

Think like Thomas Edison, who said, "I have not failed. I've just found 10,000 ways that won't work." If he had given up after finding 500 ways that didn't work, he wouldn't have invented the lightbulb. He changed the world by having the mindset that failure is progress.

Think of how you can change your life and in turn extend your life. **Let your mind wander to how good it will feel when you have the energy and liveliness to impact those around you and change the world!** The road to success is not just about what works for you. Finding out what doesn't work can be just as powerful!

Take a moment to imagine your new life. Ask yourself these questions:
What does your life actually feel like when you have broken out of your cocoon and become the butterfly you were aspiring to be?

What would your first thoughts and feelings be when you wake up in the morning?

What might you be doing that day?

What are you looking forward to?

How good does it feel to have immense amounts of energy and feel good living inside your own body?

How strong and sexy do you feel?

What about when you look in the mirror for the first time that day- what are your thoughts and feelings?

What types of people are in your life?

How do they help you become a better person that contributes positively to the world?

What do you fill your days doing?

How do you take care of your emotional and physical needs?

What are your new favorite foods and things to do?

How do you feel at the end of the day knowing you have taken care of your body, mind, and spirit?

What types of thoughts and emotions do you have more often now?

I challenge you to go through the previous paragraph before falling asleep every night and imagine these things in vivid detail. This exercise is very powerful! While you imagine this as you are falling asleep, let your positive emotions become bigger and bigger as you let yourself feel happy, accomplished, successful, confident, and just celebrate your victory of becoming a healthy person who lives a healthy lifestyle! Celebrate yourself!!

What if you step out of your comfort zone and it doesn't feel very comfortable? What if you step out and it feels overwhelming and challenging to keep it up? Congratulations! This means that you are on the road to success. Feeling uncomfortable and challenged is the definition of stepping out of your comfort zone. In fact, this is exactly how you can tell that you have done it right! The goal is to feel very uncomfortable and start to "fail" (find out what doesn't work for you). At that point, you can realize that you are doing a very good job and you are definitely and obviously taking the right actions!

This is the point when you can feel very proud of yourself and acknowledge you are on the right track every hour of the day! Give yourself an emotional pat on the back or hug. Tell someone you know who will be supportive when you want extra encouragement and acknowledgement for what you are doing! If you are going to spend money to reward yourself now and then, instead of spending it on going out or on decadent food, treat yourself with things you love. For example, a massage, a membership to your favorite new yoga studio, new workout clothes, golf clubs, a blender that makes it easier to make healthy green shakes, or a weekend at the beach or mountains. This is the time to really take care of yourself and acknowledge doing what most people are not brave enough to do.

Consider this mindset:

It is not the critic who counts; not the man who points out how the strong man stumbles, or where the doer of deeds could have done them better. The credit belongs to the man who is actually in the arena, whose face is marred by dust and sweat and blood; who strives valiantly; who errs, who comes short again and again, because there is no effort without error and shortcoming; but who does actually strive to do the deeds; who knows great enthusiasms, the great devotions; who spends himself in a worthy cause; who at the best knows in the end the triumph of high achievement, and who at the worst if he fails, at least fails while daring greatly, so that his place shall never be with those cold and timid souls who neither know victory nor defeat. (Excerpt from Theodore Roosevelt's speech "Citizenship In A Republic", delivered at the Sorbonne, in Paris, France on April 23, 1910).

Now that you are willing to take a risk and step out of your comfort zone, you may wonder how exactly to go about taking your first steps? If you were able to get ahold of and read this book, you most likely have the ability to learn and develop your healthy living skills. Information is everywhere--on the internet, books, classes, peers, and mentors. I greatly respect your ability to research and decide on your own path towards living a long, healthy life.

Since I often get questioned about specific actions to take to live a healthy life, I will provide a brief outline of how to go about researching and deciding on habits and a lifestyle that will give you your desired body, energy level, and make you deeply content.

First of all, develop an interest in health topics so that you eventually become the expert in knowing what is best for YOU. Get into the habit of letting health-related articles, shows, conversations, and locations catch your eye and explore! Follow social media pages that promote healthy living (mind, body, and spirit) and read articles to learn more. Unfollow things and people that do not nurture your heart, body, and mind. Think of the type of body you would like to live in. Explore the types of information that people who have created that body and lifestyle feed their minds with every day. For example, if you would like to build a lot more muscle and gain weight, read articles about weight lifting and start to notice what people with your ideal body type are interested in and do. If you would like to significantly reduce your overall weight and are not interested in adding much muscle, read articles on success stories and how people developed that lifestyle. There will be different types of articles and people that you will follow depending on your specific goals.

Secondly, Surround yourself as much as possible with healthy people and learn from them. You may know a friend or someone at work who manages to live the healthy kind of lifestyle you would like to live. If you would like, let them know that you admire and look up to what they have created in their lives. They will likely be happy to hear you acknowledge this. This will also help your unconscious mind know that you admire and have good feelings towards successful people (in the fitness arena and otherwise). Letting yourself have good feelings towards and acknowledge those who already have what you have is extremely healthy for YOU. The reason is that it releases you to also succeed while still loving yourself. Think about it- if you secretly hate successful people, when you become successful, will you be able to fully love and celebrate yourself, too? Or will you sabotage yourself and wonder why? ALWAYS celebrate your successes and the successes of others.

Ask a friend, acquaintance, or co-worker if they would be willing to coach or mentor you for a few weeks to steer you in the right direction. You might tag along with them at the gym or get lunch with them and notice and copy what they do and eat. Notice how they manage their stress levels and energy throughout the day while still staying healthy. Become curious and ask them lots of questions. Most healthy people wish there were more healthy people in the world and will be happy to share their lifestyle with you and have a friend supporting their own healthy habits. You can hire people to do this as well, depending on the intensity you desire. For example, you can hire a personal trainer, join a yoga studio (and make a habit of attending consistently), go to vegan cooking classes, or join a support group.

Creating the life you want can be done for free and is often just as successful as paying someone to do it for you. When you create support groups or friend groups who support each other in this way, you know others are depending on you and it becomes a reward in itself to show up for each other.

Follow what you are interested in and believe in yourself. Try new things! Think about it--do you enjoy ice cream? Did you know you loved ice cream when you were born? No, you never knew you loved ice cream until you tried it for the first time! There are so many healthy new things to try out there. Go find some new, delicious things to eat, activities, people to befriend, and ways to change the world. Live a new adventure every day. You will never know what wonderful things can take your life to the next level without first being open and trying it out! There was that first day of your life when you opened your mouth and decided to try something new. You ended up loving it. If you never tried it, you might never have known what it was like!

Let me tell you a secret--life isn't about reaching one accomplishment and then relaxing and being self centered after that is all met. Life is a lifestyle of enjoying being the best person you can be, renewing your commitment to live according to your values and ideals, learning how to have a happier and richer life and help others do so, too. Enjoy the process of repeatedly devouring your cocoon!

Chapter 6

Become Bulletproof

A person who never made a mistake never tried anything new. -Albert Einstein

I've missed more than 9000 shots in my career. I've lost almost 300 games. 26 times I've been trusted to take the game winning shot and missed. I've failed over and over and over again in my life. And that is why I succeed.
-Michael Jordan

Fall down seven times, get up eight.
-Japanese Proverb

Have you ever felt so weighed down and defeated that you wonder if you can ever pick yourself up again? Are you overwhelmed with life, dealing with chaos, loss, and stress?

Have you wondered lately how you can ever really make a lasting internal change to lose weight for good? Guess what? You actually have a great advantage in life.

Have you heard that life is not about what happens to you but how you react to it?

Try flipping the switch in your mind today. Creating this new mindset can literally change your life: It may or may not be true that many things have happened in your life that you did not have control over in the past. The important question is: Do you realize how much power you actually have now? Don't let your past experiences fool you! Your current amount of power is extraordinary regardless of your past.

If you are an adult with most basic freedoms, you have immense control over your health and fitness. Think about it- when everything in life feels chaotic and out of control in the world, economy, relationships... anything external, you can still have control over your own health and body.

When you feel trapped or as though you have little or no control over the bad circumstances in your life, think of this: You may not have control of certain things in your life right now. However, you have control over how you react to setbacks and difficult times. When the circumstances in your life seem uncontrollably stressful, one thing to always keep in mind is that you do have complete control of how you treat your body with food, exercise, water, supplements, and sleep. You will almost always have control over these basic things that affect your health and body no matter what other circumstances you may face.

You can go for a walk, do pushups and stretches, decide what to eat, drink lots of water, take supplements your body needs, and focus on getting enough sound sleep because these are the basic things that you can control. If you have small children or certain types of jobs, getting adequate sleep may be a challenge in this phase of your life. However, if you focus on the things you can control and do the absolute best you can to manage your life, you will see amazing results. Also, some people have found that when they learn how to eat, drink, exercise, and take supplements if needed, their bodies start to need less rest.

If you have gone through the worst of times, you now deserve to create and live in the best of times. Love your body now and create a healthy and energetic body you love to live in. You deserve it! Let the past failures and storms of life you have been through only bring you immense power and wisdom, making you bulletproof!

Recognize how your cocoon used to protect you as you were growing and becoming bulletproof. Your wings are now free! Now focus on enjoying such a free feeling. This step is the most powerful for most people. It can make the difference between sticking to a diet for a week and changing your body for a lifetime. It is what helps turn your perceived weaknesses into success.

Think ahead with me right now to what is usually you weakest point in the week. What usually triggers you to eat, drink, or do unhealthy things? Is it a certain time of day? Is it after dealing with a certain type of person? How do you feel about yourself at that time? Aside from eating, what do you really need? How do you usually respond? Does your response really feed what you need at your deepest level of being?

What would be the best and most nurturing way to respond to your own needs when you are at your weakest point? Think of a good game plan for you to take care of yourself in a healthy way next time this happens. For example, if you usually feel the most stressed on the way home from work and are tempted to stop by a drive thru, take action before you leave from work!

Grab a few nuts, your favorite snack or fruit, a warm or cold healthy drink within the hour before you leave or when you get into the car on the way home so that you make it home for a delicious and fulfilling healthy meal instead of stopping on the way for junk food.

You can call a friend or family member who is a good listener on the way home from work and tell them about your day. Take a walk at a park, a yoga class, or stop by the gym on the way home to avoid traffic. Schedule a massage, do some yard work or gardening after work, and listen to your favorite music! Treat yourself well and nurture yourself by doing this. It is actually a very generous thing to do because when you take care of your own health first, you will have even more energy and motivation. Your increased health will help you have more energy to give towards you loved ones, not to mention a longer and healthier life so that they don't have to lose you early or worry about your health. You will also have more to give to the world by treating yourself well because you will have more vitality to focus on your life's mission and ultimately make the world a better place!

Remember to speak kind and appreciative thoughts to yourself throughout the day, being grateful that you have the wisdom to navigate through situations that used to be stressful for you.

Another good way to change your thinking and feeling patterns is by listening to music or speakers who make you happy, grateful, and that make you think about something you are looking forward to instead of dwelling on a situation that brings you down. You have more control over your life and health than you realize! Use it and make it fun!

Do you know why cats purr? Most people think that they purr because they are already feeling blissful and content. Did you know that they also purr when they are scared or in pain? It is something that they do that helps them feel better whether or not they are already in this feel-good state. We can learn from cats and do the same thing! Not literally of course. Start to notice what you are doing when you feel really good. How does your body feel? What emotions are you experiencing? What thoughts are you thinking? What do you say to yourself when you first wake up or as you are falling asleep? What kind of music did you listen to? Who did you talk to and what did you talk about? What activities do you do? How are you feeling about yourself and your life?

Make an inner "note" of these feelings and practice it. Practice feeling these feelings at all times throughout the day. It is a learned skill, so it may not come easy at first. Keep practicing until you get really good at changing how you feel regardless of what is going on around you! "Purr" to yourself throughout the day and remember to do these things not only when you are feeling good, but when you are scared or in pain and need a "purr" to soothe yourself.

Learning how to change our emotional and physical state may be the most powerful skill in the world that a person can learn! Learning how to create and change our feelings instead of reacting to feelings can completely change the course of our lives and help us meet any goal we decide on!

As you know, our past "failures" propel us even faster towards goals. Think about it- the more failures a person has in their past, the further along on in the journey towards the goal they are! Having made it through many past "failures" actually provides an advantage! We know what to expect and how to prepare better this time. We know what it takes emotionally, socially, mentally, and spiritually and have the ability to visualize most clearly what success is.

Past pain and hard times are now victory flags. It has made you so much stronger and wiser. You know that the worst is over and that since you have made it through the darkest times, it can only get brighter and better from here on out!

Everyone has hard times. Think about it- the most admired and successful people in history have not been born into an easy life. They went through the most difficult times. The difference is that they had a different mindset and their perseverance and actions made them a great success.

Abraham Lincoln is famously known as saying, "I will prepare, and someday my chance will come." By the age of 50, Abraham Lincoln had lost his job, failed in business, lost his sweetheart to death, had a nervous breakdown, was defeated for speaker, nomination for congress, land officer, and U.S. senate twice and Vice President. Then, one day before his 52nd birthday, he became the President of the United States. Its a good thing he didn't quit after his first few defeats! The same lesson is here for us. Don't give up. Consider every failure a stepping stone to success. There is a life purpose for each one of us. Don't quit too soon! Just let go of your own time table and keep learning and revising, enjoying the journey!

A class I was once in was given a fascinating assignment one evening. We could not leave the room or go home for the night until we have tried to sell our product and been rejected by at least 14 of our peers! I have a strong drive to do an excellent job and succeed in whatever I put my mind to, but this situation was socially uncomfortable for me, so staying in that room and doing this assignment was very challenging. Nevertheless, I followed the directions and did not leave until I was rejected about 12 times. At that point, there were no other new people in the room to sell to (most people gave up and left early because failing was so uncomfortable)! I ended up coming in second place out of about 100 people for number of sales that weekend just because I stuck to it and didn't give up on my assignment to fail 14 times. I had never sold a product before in my life. I did not do anything extraordinary that evening except I failed more than anyone else, resulting in success.

I realized then that when I saw failure and rejection as part of the process of success, it did the trick for me to keep going and gave me momentum. Sounds strange but it is a strategic psychological principle that worked!

Perseverance and success is a journey and "failures" are roadsigns telling you that you are going the right direction! This is how you become bulletproof. Roadblocks become victory flags. Let your past storms bring you power and wisdom, rather than pain and self doubt. Recognize what your cocoon used to do for you and how your wings are now free!

Select your thoughts carefully. Focus on the things you are thankful for and what you want more of. Life is too short to worry about the not so great things. Focus your thoughts and energy on what you want. Also, remember to treat yourself the way you would want someone you love to be treated. Take care of your health and your body. Your body is a good support system for your mind and spirit and vice versa. You are a magnificent treasure.

Chapter 7

Your Soul's Deepest Cravings

Take care of your body. It's the only place you have to live. -Jim Rohn

The intuitive mind is a sacred gift and the rational mind a faithful servant. We have created a society that honors the servant and has forgotten the gift - Albert Einstein

Radical healing takes radical feeling
-Daphne Erhart

What does carrying excess weight or being tired and unhealthy give to you? Believe it or not, there may be some not so obvious "benefits". Has it helped you feel protected from sexual or jealous attention that might make you scared or embarrassed? Has remaining unfit provided you with an excuse for not doing things that would scare you? Has being unhealthy kept your loved ones' attention and prompted them to express their care and love for you more? Has it kept you in the familiar feeling of feeling bad about yourself, which is familiar and comfortable?

Does carrying extra weight help you avoid something that might be scary or uncomfortable? Does overeating give you a feeling of fulfillment that you don't get elsewhere in your life? Does it help you not feel so bored, frustrated, or lonely? What emotions may you be "stuffing down" with excess food or drinks (or any legal or illegal substances for that matter) instead of dealing with them in healthy ways so that you are empowered, healthy, happy, and utterly content in your life?

Do you know what you truly want? What makes you feel blissful and fulfilled? Begin this new habit today: Be in a state of mind where you allow yourself to recognize your own true motives and needs. Treat yourself as you would a young, innocent child. Be completely accepting, kind, and nurturing towards yourself! Once you truly know and do what is best for you, you have more to give to others and may already be on your way to solve things that were formerly problems in your life. This particular step of recognizing what you are really craving and giving yourself (and your soul) what it really needs deep down is a very individual process. Let your mind wander and meditate on your real cravings and desires. Be kind to yourself and nurture yourself. Allow the real issues start to come up instead of stuffing them down.

When uncomfortable thoughts and feelings come up for you, let yourself fully experience it. You can handle it! You will live through feeling your feelings and thinking your thoughts! The worst thing you can do for yourself is pretend your thoughts and feelings aren't there, no matter how horrible they seem. Let yourself fully feel them and then let it go. Otherwise, how can you release what you deny is even there?

If processing these things with another person helps you, make sure you accept support when you want it. If for any reason it is especially difficult for you or if trauma surfaces, make sure you have the help of a professional psychologist or therapist to get through this phase. Professionals can help you process these things and help you move on in your life. Just make sure to choose a professional who does help you move towards your goals. It might be comforting to know that it is impossible to have an extreme emotion forever. No matter how sad you are, your body eventually stops crying, your body and emotions shift (whether slowly or quickly), and at some point, you are finally able to heal and move on. The thing that triggers the difficult emotions (e.g. loss or grief) may still be there, but you will survive and it is possible to move past sadness, grief, anger, or any other difficult emotion. Remember that emotions are like clouds in the sky. You can notice them, acknowledge and fully experience them, and then let them float on by and dissipate. You always have the choice whether or not to act on an emotion. Thoughts and emotions may float in and out of your experience. What you decide to do with them is fully your responsibility. Choose wisely. Choose actions that will make the lives of both you and others better!

As you start to become more of an expert at detecting what unhealthy living previously did for you, learn to thank yourself, love yourself, and take some kind of action to immediately fulfill whatever desires and cravings come up. For example, if you realize you are actually lonely, call or text someone immediately to set up a time to do something with them (in person). Be aware of who you contact and make sure you connect with someone who is closest to the kind of "emotionally healthy" companionship you are wanting. Or if you are really craving some excitement, look up a meet-up or any type of group (same day if possible), who is doing something new and exciting!

Are you usually feeling relaxed and peaceful, or stressed and anxious? Stress and relaxation are very powerful aspects of healthy living and weight loss. As you may have noticed in your personal life, increased stress leads to weight gain and health problems while proper relaxation and rest leads to healthy weight, metabolism, and body processes. Increased stress raises the cortisol levels, which may naturally make your body hang on to fat, not to mention the tendency to overeat when stressed out. Stress can be distracting and you may not realize just how much food you are putting into your body. This is why it is a good idea to create a ritual to center yourself, relax your body, and be in a grateful and calm emotional state when eating. Choosing different types of foods, eating habits, timing meals, snacks, and amounts of different types of foods can also help manage stress, moods, and promote healthy weight.

Give yourself alone time every day to get in touch with your feelings, what you truly desire more of in your life, and what will make you feel more fulfilled and content. Let yourself realize in a safe and supportive environment what your worst fears are, what you may be protecting yourself from, and what you feel you need. Be unconditionally loving and accepting of yourself as you let yourself become aware of these things. Everyone in this world has gone through different experiences and has their own path. Everyone's experiences and individual challenges are different. Accept everything that comes up for you. Nurture yourself daily and accept what you truly want and need. You are worthy of doing all of these things for yourself every day. Let go of the past disappointments and move on. Recognize your true needs, past hurts and traumas, and let yourself become aware of what kind of treatment and environment would help you fully heal in the quickest and most complete way possible. Finally, start to take action to provide this healing environment for yourself.

For example, are you craving your favorite comfort food? Deep down, what are you expecting to feel like after you have eaten it?

What is the real thing you want?   A real friend to talk to who will validate and accept you? True, unconditional love? Quality nutritious food that may be a bit more expensive but worth it for your body? Fun exercise? Sunshine? Quiet time for yourself? Self confidence? Excitement? To feeling accomplished? To feel like you really made a difference in someone's life? Feeling truly valued and loved through your connections to other people? Let yourself become more and more aware each day to your soul's deepest cravings.

Keep practicing your new expertise of recognizing and fulfilling what you need. Before long, you will have developed a very powerful skill in this area that will give your whole life a boost in the right direction! Keep moving step by step and before long you will be celebrating your accomplishments!

Recognize and take ownership for your true needs and cravings and meet them so that you get what you want in every area, including health and fitness.

We are built to live a life full of love and joy and connection. **There is something at the core of all of us that is able to sense when that need to live a meaningful life full of real, loving connections is fulfilled. We know deep down when we are living our purpose in this world or not.** Have you ever been around many people yet did not really feel connected to anyone? During those moments, do you know what you really want and crave or do you just have a general sense of discomfort, boredom, sadness, or deep craving to do something that changes your physical or emotional state (such as eating)?

Did you feel wanted and unconditionally loved growing up? Do you feel that way now? If not, what types of connections do you want to create? You are not alone- there are tons of people just like you throughout this planet who also crave the same thing and who - just like you - are capable of deeply caring for and connecting with another person. We just tend to get into the habit of being what society calls "appropriate". Believe it or not, if you smile at the person next to you in line at the store, express empathy with a stranger, and are willing to be vulnerable first, you will likely start to develop deeply meaningful and satisfying relationships with others, leading to more feelings of fulfillment and satisfaction. It takes practice, and now that you know where to start, you can continue to develop this ability to connect with others.

If you are lucky enough to have experienced unconditional love at some time in your life, you probably know how life-changing the experience is. Let me tell you a story about my abuelita (great-grandmother). I've heard so many stories about her fearlessness and this one demonstrates the kind of deep unconditional love I'm talking about. Most men in her family including her husband and most brothers were killed during a civil war in the country of Honduras. One of my favorite stories is about her immense love for her son. She raised four daughters, her granddaughter (my mother), and also adopted and raised a boy as her own.

One day during that civil war, armed men came to where she was hiding and demanded her to hand over the boy so that they could kill him. Instead of doing what they demanded or freezing in fear like most people would do, she quickly told her newly adopted son to hide under the bed, then blocked the way, telling them that if they intended to kill her son, they would have to kill her first to get by her. They decided not to kill her and consequently they did not kill her son, letting both of them live.

This story was told to me many years ago with such devotion and love by her own son. As you can imagine, witnessing her willingness to risk her life for him and experiencing first hand how much she really loved him changed his life forever. As he told me this story many years ago, it became clear that his love, dedication, and passion for life stemmed from being raised with such immense love. Witnessing such an act made him feel deeply loved and he was devoted to her for the rest of his life. Can you imagine seeing the person who loves you the most, ready to die for you at a moment's notice?

Do you recognize and know what you want to experience in your life spiritually? I believe in God. I also respect your spiritual beliefs and experiences regardless of whether or not they are similar or different than mine. Regardless of your spiritual beliefs, I hope you will take some moments right now to acknowledge your soul's deepest cravings and consider these questions. Do you have a longing for a deeper connection with God or a higher power? Would feeling more spiritually connected fulfill something that your soul deeply desires? Would you feel more purposeful and peaceful? This realization and connection regardless of how much we do or don't fully understand what is bigger than us can be life-changing and profoundly meaningful.

I feel incredibly lucky because I have personally realized there is a higher power who is Love and receiving that love has changed my ability to live openly in life with an internal knowledge that I am loved by the Maker of the Universe. God is love and I believe that all people are loved even more than we can even imagine. Deeply realizing that we are deeply loved unconditionally is completely healing, fulfilling, and life changing. This immense unconditional love for us is the food for our souls that we naturally crave. This pure, unconditional love is healing, and when we love each other and are open to receiving this kind of love, it is immensely healing to our hearts and bodies as well.

I saw this quote the other day and it looked like it was intended as part of a decoration for a child's bedroom:

> Before you were conceived, I wanted you.
> Before you were born, I loved you.
> Before you were here an hour,
> I would die for you.
> This is the miracle of love.
> —Maureen Hawkins

At first glance, the quote touched my heart because it is such a sweet thought that a parent would feel this love toward their child even before they were conceived. But as I thought about it more, it touched me on an even deeper level and I started to wonder if Maureen Hawkins realized she was echoing God's powerful love for us.

"Before I formed you in the womb I knew you",
and, "I have loved you with an everlasting
love" (Jeremiah 1:5; 31:3).

Throughout our lives, when we experience deep
heartaches and stress, this experience can lead
to a flawed concepts of what love is. Painful
human experiences can make it more of a
challenge to imagine the reality of true
unconditional love for us or even be in a state of
mind where we can experience or accept this
kind of love when it does come our way. But it
doesn't have to be like this! Realizing and
experiencing pure and powerful love gives us so
many things including healthy self-esteem,
energy to love others unconditionally, motivation
and purpose in life, and a deep sense of peace
and joy.

Being completely and unconditionally loved is
life-changing regardless of status, financial or
educational success, popularity, and self-
sufficiency. Everyone has the capacity to love
and be loved. Everyone is born with the ability to
have genuine and deeply loving and fulfilling
connections with other people. Instead of filling
an unacknowledged sense of emptiness with
things, food, substances, possessions,
accomplishments, etc. Become aware of what

94

you really want and need. Let yourself be open, genuinely connect with others, and be receptive and vulnerable to receive unconditional love.

Also practice being grateful, loving, and appreciative for your own magnificent body right now. It is almost impossible to maintain a positive change in healthy living if it is based on negativity or self-hatred. Focusing on that ugly inner feeling of self-loathing creates more difficult internal feelings, which can trigger the desire to substitute the terrible feelings with food or something else. Be careful not to create a feeling or belief that you will later want to stuff down with food! If you come from a place of gratefulness and love for your own body and what your body has been able to do to sustain you over the years, there will be less negativity to deal with by overeating.

What is your definition of forgiveness? Ironically, forgiving someone who wronged you in the past gives you freedom and power! Do you agree or disagree? Some people feel that forgiving someone means they are saying it is alright that they were wronged. That is not forgiveness. Forgiveness is not letting yourself be harmed, taken advantage of, or in any way saying it was ever ok that you or someone else was wronged.

Forgiveness happens inside of you only. It is mainly for you to have freedom, empowerment, and liberation. Forgiveness will give you more power, peace, and the ability to have deep happiness and love again even though you were harmed or wronged in the past. It is not letting what the other person did to you fester inside your soul and become a disease that eats up the joy in your life. Forgiving, holding someone accountable for their actions, and creating healthy boundaries can happen all at once.

At first glance, it can look like forgiveness requires vulnerability to the very person who hurt you but in reality, it gives you untouchable strength! **If you are able to forgive the other person, smile open-heartedly again to life's experiences even though you have been severely harmed in the past, imagine the strength and power you must have that they were not able to take from you!** The perpetrator will have to deal with whatever comes their way and their hurtful behavior towards others will never be condoned, yet they have less and less power as soon as their victims refuse to let it stick with them anymore. A perpetrator should never be allowed to continue, however. Never confuse forgiveness with letting yourself be harmed again. If someone harmed you or someone you know, make sure you keep appropriate boundaries (and if necessary, notify authorities) so that it does not happen again. If they attempt to do it again, be strong and put a stop to it immediately and do not let it spoil your day if at all possible!

Be kind to yourself as you accept any self-realizations or memories that come up throughout this process of exploring your true wants and needs. There are so many things that can come to the surface that it is impossible to ever write down all of the possible combinations of issues, feelings, and processes someone might go through. We all have unique life experiences, predispositions, personalities, and personal desires. Everyone attempts to fulfill these desires and take care of themselves in different ways.

In a way, overeating or any "maladaptive" habit formed was once a first attempt to recognize and take care of oneself. Everyone does the best they can at any given time in their lives, so you can thank yourself for recognizing your own needs and caring, nurturing, and attempting to fulfill one or some of your deepest needs. Realize that your unique way of attempting to fulfill your soul's deepest desires is based on pure intentions. Feel free to explore this with a professional if something comes up that seems unmanageable to deal with alone.

I know an amazing and beautiful mother who became overweight after an awful betrayal and abuse at the hands of her ex-husband. After a couple of years of being out of the situation and reflecting on it, she discovered that one of the reasons she hangs on to the weight is her fear of being available for love again and also her fear of being pursued again only for her physical attractiveness. She didn't truly believe she could protect herself in such a deeply involved emotional situation again.   She went through years of emotional, physical, and sexual abuse without even realizing it was abuse at that time. At the beginning of the relationship, she was trusting, loving, and open. After many years of abuse coupled with not knowing how to safely get out of the situation with her children, she was severely and repeatedly hurt and taken advantage of over the course of many years, resulting in deep heartache and making the next few years of her life unbelievably difficult in many ways.

She worked hard as a single mother to support her children and was not interested in being available to romantic relationships with men because in her mind, that meant risking almost every aspect of her life again. Finally, she came to the realization that in her course of healing, she could trust herself to make wise and emotionally safe decisions regarding romantic relationships. This is not necessarily as easy as it sounds to someone who has experienced extreme trauma over the course of several years. It is a process that she has already started that includes practicing, asking the opinions of loved ones who share her values, forgiving, healing (partially by letting herself experience other healthy and unconditionally loving relationships), being able to detect interpersonal patterns more quickly than she used to, trusting her own feelings and reactions, and trusting her ability to put up appropriate boundaries if or when the time arises, and much, much more. It is a step by step process to go through. She has already lost 20 pounds and kept it off, and let herself be open to a new relationship and real love. She is also now happily re-married!

There was another man who grew up very poor. He was homeless at times, living with his mother and siblings out of a car when he was very young. At times, he didn't know where his next meal would come from. At every opportunity to eat, he quickly learned to eat as much as he could to "stock up", since he didn't know how long he would have to wait until the next meal. Any kind of food was welcome, and the more dense in calories, the better it felt to eat it after being in starvation mode for hours or even days at times. In addition to this way of learning to "hoard" food for survival at such a young age, this man's happiest memories where he felt the most secure and loved as a child was when his mom would bring chips and candy bars from the grocery store and together with his siblings, they would eat and laugh together. His subconscious mind associates junk food and candy bars with deeply comforting and happy feelings. As you can imagine, his personal challenge as a grown man now creating new, healthy habits are different than someone who grew up with three square meals and memories of tomato soup by the fireplace as their comfort food.

What if there was a "reset" button we could push to undo all of the negative programming in our lives? What if we could then create a detailed picture of how we want to act and feel in our daily lives so that our way of being is inherently healthy, even down to what and how we eat and take care of our bodies? The timing it takes to "reset" is different from person to person, so please be patient with yourself and realize that taking the next step (whatever that may be for you) and moving at any speed today is much better than waiting until later to start on this journey.

During this process, please open your mind and heart to reach deep within as you re-program your way of being. The more open, honest, and vulnerable you are willing to be, the better results you will get. You will start to notice ways of interacting, feeling, and moving throughout your life change. You are the author and artist of your life and your being. Let's form new ways of living by consciously starting some new habits and releasing the unhelpful ones.

Get into the habit of giving yourself some alone time every morning. Make this a priority. You were made to shine. Embrace every part of you that makes up who you are. Love and accept yourself completely. If you have a son or daughter, think of the immense unconditional love you have for them. You are probably able to see their strengths and weaknesses, their faults and talents. You are able to accept them completely and deeply love them and nurture them so that they have the best life possible.

Practice this on yourself. It will make you even more capable to do this with others.

Everyone is born as a unique work of art. However, if you judge all people as having to fit into a particular mold or style of art, they may feel they don't measure up when in reality they could be an unrecognized and undetected Picasso! You are extremely special and amazing just the way you are! Realize that you were never made to be exactly like anyone else. What makes you different makes you strong and beautiful. Don't worry about what others think of you. Practice loving yourself and valuing your own opinion of yourself more than anyone else's. You are the biggest expert on what you want and need.

Above all, make sure you are loving and respecting yourself first. Make sure you are wanting to be healthy so that you can have a fuller, more enjoyable life. If you are going to release excess weight, dig deep to find the true and loving reason you are doing this. For example, decide that you will feel more blissful and content walking around with a healthy body because it will feel good and because you want to live a long life doing things you love. An example of what not to do would be trying to lose weight so that you will be loved more by your partner or so that you will feel accepted or liked by someone else. Enjoy your personal experience of living a healthy, fully expressed life.

Enjoy this allegory:
There was a young woman who had always wanted to be an artist. Ever since she was a little girl, she had beautiful dreams of colorful paintings she would like to create someday after she became a talented artist. When she would wake up from her dream, she wanted to recreate her dream so badly that she would analyze the painting she had dreamed of and take detailed notes on these dreams in her journal so that she could one day create what she saw in her mind. She believed that if she worked hard enough and made herself think it through to the tiniest detail, she would someday have the talent to replicate these things she dreamed of. The young woman picked up a paintbrush once in a while, but would not invest in good paintbrushes until she became an expert. She didn't let herself set aside any time for painting since she believed she needed to finish school, where she would learn the proper techniques to perfect her craft. She mentioned her dream of becoming a painter to a friend once, but her friend had never even seen her paint and encouraged her to give up the dream and pursue a more secure job.

One day, the young woman was diagnosed with a terminal disease and for the first time in her life she realized how precious her time was. She suddenly got so tired of dreaming of these beautiful things and not painting them in real life as she longed to do. She brought out the huge canvas she had saved up for a special occasion, bought a new set of paints, and after a long night's sleep filled with beautiful dreams of paintings, she decided to just spend the day painting whatever her heart created without planning it out first. She decided to do what she loved to do because of the enjoyment she would get out of the process of creating it, rather than making sure the end product was perfect.

After the day was over, she stepped away from her new painting to get her first glimpse of the entire canvas. She was astonished by the beauty of her new painting! She had not expected it to come out well, since her goal was her enjoyment rather than using perfect techniques. She was shocked that she LOVED it even more than she loved the paintings in her dreams! She saw that the combinations of vibrant colors and energetic composition of the piece was something she could have never created if she had stifled herself by calculating every stroke of paint. It was even more beautiful than what she had dreamed about and she had more fun than she had imagined she could have!

Somehow the process of letting herself enjoy her deepest desire and talent healed her body, too. She realized that letting go and enjoying the process rather than focusing on being certain that the outcome was perfect was the most liberating, fun, and empowering feeling ever! She dedicated the rest of her life to letting herself be the fully expressed, shining artist that she always had been inside by focusing on the journey, not rigidly forcing herself to conform to society's expectations.

Chapter 8

Drop the Deadweight
and Create Your Community

When a flower doesn't bloom you fix the environment in which it grows, not the flower. -Alexander Den Jeijer

You are the average of the five people you spend the most time with. -Jim Rohn

Walk with the wise and become wise, for a companion of fools suffers harm. -Proverbs 13:20

Choose Your Mentors and Role Models

Who do you choose to look up to as a mentor? Choose to look up to those "bigger" than you whom you admire. Choose those who are "experts in their field" or have developed an aspect(s) of themselves that you want to be most like. Be specific and consciously choose who you look up to.

Here are three things to look for in finding a successful role model or mentor:

1. Is it obvious that this person lives the life they say that they value? You should of course choose a mentor and role model who has already met the goal you are working towards, not someone who just talks about it. Sometimes this takes some time to find out how they really live their life. Talking the talk is easy. Walking the walk is the true challenge. Watch what people do more than what they say.

2. Secondly, observe how exactly have they met their health and fitness goals. Ask some honest questions. Is their lifestyle something that can be kept up for a long, healthy, lifetime while promoting happiness? Do they use drastic measures that can't be kept up over the long term? Do they have to regularly use caffeine or other supplements that are unhealthy or harmful to use over the long term? Do they motivate themselves with negative thinking, adhere to a very restrictive diet, or excessive exercise that would be almost impossible (or harmful) to replicate long term? Or do they live happy, fun, and

wholesome lives incorporating eating, exercise, sleeping, drinking, and awesome relationships that will sustain their inner and outer health and radiance for the rest of their lives?

3. Does your potential mentor encourage a rewarding lifestyle change or is it a prescribed diet or exercise regimen that is implemented for a quick fix by a certain date? Maintaining ideal fitness goals long term is a bigger challenge than initially reaching the goal because it requires a long term lifestyle change to stay at your goal indefinitely. It is much easier to restrict or take drastic measure for short term results. Maintaining it long term takes a solid, lasting inner change. Learn to notice what will help you maintain a healthy life for the rest of your life and only accept a mentor who matches you in this area.

Let yourself notice successful mentors and their lifestyles. Think critically about which parts of their lifestyle you will adopt. Just because someone is successful in one area of their life, it doesn't mean all aspects of the person are worth modeling or imitating. Also, remember that as you become successful in creating and maintaining a healthy lifestyle, you may soon be a role model and mentor to others. In fact, there is always someone who sees where you are as successfully living their next step. You may be modeled and admired without even knowing it right now!

Here is one more thing to consider. Be careful about who you put on a pedestal. Mentors and role models are great. Especially when they have been successful in the aspect of life you are working to improve. However, remember that nobody is perfect! As you get to know them, you may notice that they make mistakes. If and when they make a mistake, remember that they are human and dealing with their mistake is their own responsibility. Don't spend too much energy judging the situation or making meaning out of it to apply into your own life. Their actions are their own responsibility and have nothing to do with you. Appreciate all you can learn and imitate the good aspects of their lifestyle while staying aware to the parts that you want to leave behind.

When I was a 19 year-old college student, I thought I wanted to be a nurse. By my third year of college, I had completed all prerequisite courses and had already spent a year in a top notch nursing school doing hospital rotations. I had already put a lot of time and effort into this goal, yet the more nursing experience I completed, the clearer it became to me that I did not want to work as a nurse for the rest of my life. I pursued it far enough to know that it was not a good personality fit. I started to know deep down that although I wanted to help people and value health, it became very clear that year that being a psychologist was what I wanted to do with all my heart. I realized that at my core, working as a psychologist to help and heal was the best fit for my innate abilities and interests.

I took a leap at that point and decided that even though I had put in years of preparation to be a nurse, I knew myself better than anyone else and knew that I was meant to be a psychologist.

I met with my academic advisor and told her my plans to change my major in the middle of my third year of university. I explained to her that I wanted to change directions and work towards becoming a psychologist instead of a nurse. I was very shy and tender-hearted when I was younger and although I was very certain of what I was meant to do, I'm sure I did not come across as confident. It took all the courage I had to go to my advisor's office and tell her I wanted to switch majors.

Even though I was more of a quiet listener rather than an outgoing advice-giver back then, I had enough wisdom to know that I knew better than anyone else in the world what I wanted and what my "purpose" was. I knew deep down that I had what it takes to help people as a psychologist. When I told her I was going to be a psychologist instead of a nurse, I clearly remember how startled and disappointed she looked. She paused, and then gave me an almost pitiful smile saying, "but Daphne, you know you have to actually talk to people to be a psychologist"? She was a chatty person and clearly believed I did not have what it takes to be a psychologist because she viewed me as having a quiet, receptive personality. Little did she know that it would become one of my biggest strengths in my profession. I didn't know until I reached graduate school that I had a natural ability to listen and then quickly and accurately detect what a person needs to create movement in their lives. Making sure I fully understand people's emotions, goals, and how to get them "unstuck" creates movement in their lives very quickly and easily. This came naturally to me because I didn't view being a psychologist as giving advice without fully understanding the other person first. Making sure I fully understand a person and their situation is an asset. Knowing exactly where they are "stuck", and then using my expertise to guide them to where they wanted to go is a strength.   I'm so glad I listened to my instincts about what I was capable of doing and did not cave in to what someone I had put on a pedestal thought was best for me.

Sometimes I wonder what my life would have been like if I had taken other people's advice and didn't follow what I knew I was naturally good at. What would have happened if I had not listened to myself and instead, tried to conform to what other people told me to do with my life?

It is wise to have mentors and role models, but always think critically about what advice they give you. Listen to your own inner wisdom and self-knowledge first. Never let anyone else have power over your conscience or decisions. Always respect yourself, love yourself, and get in touch with what your heart and soul knows is best for you.

Carefully Choose Your Entourage

Do the people in your life support a healthy lifestyle or do you get off track with your fitness goals every time you spend time together? It takes energy and strength to create and maintain new lifestyle habits. Think about whether the people closest to you support and encourage your health goals even when you are feeling weak or whether they encourage you to ditch your new healthy lifestyle. Do they create more stress for you or are they a source of support?

Fair weather friends are by your side to celebrate with you when your life is wonderful, yet disappear when you need it the most. You may have also noticed that there are also people who are more than happy to be there for you when you are feeling down or not doing so great but because of their own insecurities, become unsupportive when you start to do well. You cannot control the actions of others. Your job is to be wise about who you surround yourself with. Choose people who are true friends regardless of where you are on the ups and downs of the roller coaster of life. In other words, notice who is truly supportive during both good and bad times and spend the majority of your time with those trustworthy people who truly want the best for you and whose actions reflect this. Be this type of true friend to others, too.

The people you surround yourself with makes a huge difference when it comes to your well-being and meeting your own personal goals. Think of the 5-10 people that you interact with the most every week.

Do they have similar values to you? Do they care about you unconditionally? Are they overly invested in you being successful or unsuccessful? Do you start to question yourself when you are around them? Are they threatened when you start to thrive? If your beliefs or values are not very similar, are they still respectful and supportive of your own values and goals? Make conscious decisions about who you will interact with closely in your life.

Keep those same people in mind and take note of their attitudes, beliefs, habits, and decisions regarding how they live. Are they living a life that is congruent with your values and goals? If not, are they actively working to make their lives better? It is ok to help people and be on a journey together. Just remember that the habits, attitudes, and overall lifestyle of those we are closest to greatly influence us and can propel us towards our goals faster or hold us back.

No matter how strong you think you are, those we are closest to greatly influence our lives. They influence what we talk about, think about, what we spend our time doing, eating habits, and even how we feel about ourselves. For example, have you ever been around someone who sees the world as a terrible place and is sure to point all of the bad things they notice, whether it is trash on the side of the road or a belief that there is an impending disaster? Even if you were feeling positive before you met with this negative person, you may start to notice the things they point out and see the world through their eyes to some degree. Constant negativity is unhealthy and as we know, what we focus on starts to become our own reality.

Now think of the most positive and loving people you know. What do they notice and talk about when you hang out? Do you feel more empowered and happy? How do you feel in the pit of your stomach when you spend time with them? How do your chest and throat feel? Do you feel like both of you can be completely congruent when communicating without sacrificing your own integrity or positive mindset? Take note of these things and make whom you choose to spend time with a very conscious choice.

Everyone can have a "bad day" sometimes. It is your responsibility, however, to do everything you can to nurture positive and healthy relationships. When you start to notice yourself adopting a friend's bad mood, anxiety, pessimistic outlook, etc., experiment with holding your boundaries. Depending on the situation, you can choose not to spend as much time with them and/or let them in on your goals to be in charge of your thoughts and feelings as much as possible and choose peace, joy, and love in your life. Chances are, they want to feel good too, but just don't realize they have the power to choose their thoughts and emotions for the most part. Life is much more fun when we choose to be happy, healthy, and focus on the best things in life- the things we can control.

If you are not able to give a friend what they want or need at a particular time, forgive yourself for not being superman or superwoman, do only what you can while still taking care of yourself. You may have to limit the time you spend with them temporarily if it starts to wear you down.

And don't worry! You can do this while continuing to treasure and respect them.

What I've found helpful at times is that I explain in the most loving way possible that although I care about them and want to help, I am not able to give them what they need at that time. If it happens repeatedly, I respect myself and remain aware in the choices I make as much as possible.

Make a mindful choice about including supportive people in your life, choosing the right mentors for you, and forming a game plan for what to do when you feel vulnerable and without the support you need.

The funny thing about life is that you can choose your friends but you cannot usually choose your family (aside from your significant other). For this reason, some people find dealing with unsupportive family more difficult than friends because with friends, it is more acceptable to distance yourself from them if they are negative or tear you down.

Recognize that although you may take the initiative to form relationships with mentors and friends, the family you are surrounded with day in and day out have an enormous impact on your health and endeavors to make healthy changes.

If or when family or loved ones make it harder for you to stick with your new ways of living healthfully, what will you do to make sure that you remain successful? This is a question for only you to answer. You know yourself and what motivates you more than anyone else.

For example, some people find it very helpful to see this as a challenge or game, and make sure that this adversity makes them want to work harder to have independence and not be a slave to fatigue and the previously unhealthy lifestyle. Others may find it the most helpful to remember why you have decided to change and keep that in the forefront of your mind. Above all, make sure that you have made the decision based on something you deeply desire. You are not doing this for anyone else. If you are making healthy lifestyle changes for someone else or to feel more desirable or viewed differently by others, you are less likely to be successful than doing it because you want to do it for yourself.

Have you ever stopped to notice who is really supportive of you in your life? Have you ever noticed that how people interact with you is very much influenced by what you expect of them, and how you act around them? **In other words, your beliefs and expectations of others and the world make a huge difference when it comes to what you experience in return.** Your mind and actions are immensely powerful!

I've often found this concept to be true in my life. For example, when I notice and spend time dwelling on something that I don't want in my life, I usually end up receiving the very thing I dread. However, when I go into a situation with positivity, love, and acting "as if" I will get my desired result, I usually get it!

Perception is projection. In other words, how we interpret things is based on our past experiences that have taught us how to make sense of things in life. When we interpret things in a positive or negative way, it influences the situation positively or negatively. **If you are not getting what you want, keep in mind that this is just feedback for you to re-adjust what you are doing and ultimately be successful.** Try expecting good things of others and the world. If you don't already, try imagining that you love your body and that others do, too! You might notice that positive things start to happen when you start this process!

Another key is to know exactly what you want and dwell only on what you actually want. It takes self discipline to only let your mind indulge in positive thoughts. It might be a new habit you would like to develop! Our minds are constantly working, whether we realize it or not! Its important to feed our bodies, hearts and minds healthy "food" so that we can have amazingly delicious results in all aspects of our lives!

Choose people in your life carefully. Take your time wisely choosing partners and friends. Talk about your goals and growing together. Of course, you don't always have to be talking about serious things. Have fun, relax, spend quiet moments together, and share the "little" things, too. Make sure you are surrounded by people who are committed to growth, treating themselves and others with kindness and respect, and committed to becoming the best they can be. Make a conscious decision to surround yourself with other people who have similar values and goals and encourage and support you to be your best.

There is only so much you can do by yourself. Working with like-minded people to be healthy, to meet a common goal, or to change the world is so much more powerful than trying to do it alone or surrounding yourself with people who go against your goals. It's ok to lift others up along the way but be conscious of your strength and needs, never putting yourself in jeopardy. Think about it. If you don't sustain your own momentum, how will you be able to lift others up? Make sure that you feel strong and supported before you start to let others lean on you. Never try to give to others more than the inner resources you have within yourself at a given time. Your ability to support others remains strong when you are fully supported and your momentum is up. If you are running low on fuel, fill up before giving your last drops away. It will help everyone involved be successful in the long run.

It only makes sense that people try to work in their best self-interest. Remembering that everyone does the best they can at a given time can help you avoid emotional pain and feeling hurt when people you love do things that hurt your feelings. Take nothing personally. Someone who is behaving in a destructive or unsupportive way may simply be doing the best they can in a given situation. This does not mean that you are obligated to sacrifice your own well-being. Just be aware and then decide whether or not to take what they say or do to heart. This will do wonders to your own well-being and ability to meet your own needs.

Relationships are immensely powerful in their ability to make your life peaceful or stressful, adaptive or maladaptive, successful or a struggle, healthy or unhealthy. If you are doing your absolute best, what the people closest to you are doing makes a difference. If they are constantly (whether they know it or not) pulling you down or nudging you even more towards your goal, it can make or break your ability to live the kind of life you want to live. Therefore it is wise to decide what you are willing to put up with and what you welcome into your life.

Most people do not make the deliberate choice about who will share their life with them. Friends, acquaintances, and life partners are all chosen by YOU! For example, who you spent the most time within the last month was entirely your own choice. Little by little, we decide who we allow into our lives by the small choices.

These choices reveal themselves in who we allow to complain to us, who we choose to go to happy hour with, who we text or talk to every day, or what people or groups of people we seek out to develop healthy relationships.

These choices are not set in stone. As long as we live, we are in a state of constant growth. We make mistakes and grow from them. We don't know the end from the beginning. That is why it is crucial to give yourself some grace and love. You are always doing the best you can at any given time. If you see that you have made choices that have harmed you in the past, just move on with a smile. We can't change the past but we can change and make the right choices as soon as we are aware of them.

We all have internal "rules" that we are either aware of or unaware of that greatly influence who we end up sharing our lives with. These "rules" are influenced by our values and beliefs about what is right and wrong. For example, if you have let guilt and unnecessary obligation rule your life, it may be hard for you to cut short a conversation with someone who regularly complains and negatively interprets events.

Instead of feeling guilty about setting healthy boundaries, think of it this way: That person probably doesn't realize how they are hurting themselves and those around them. Allowing them to go on is detrimental to their own health and sense of peace, not to mention the health and sense of peace of those around them and you. If you let this unhealthy cycle replicate with you, it will not help them, you, or the people you and they influence.

However, if you change the subject to something you are thankful for or mainly interact when the topics build people up, it contributes greatly to wellness. It also helps you stay in a state of love, gratefulness, and positivity, which in turn gives you more and more to share with the world.

Do not confuse mindfully choosing to be around people who have decided to have a positive mindset with ignoring someone in need of support. Even the most positive, kind, and uplifting person goes through phases where they need someone to understand and support them so they can get through their difficult time and back to their usual self. Also, make sure you truly understand someone before offering constructive criticism. It is ok to help a friend through a hard time. Over time you will find out who is truly trying to get through the hard time and who is always going through a hard time because of their negative outlook on life.

Feel free to make your decisions about who to spend time with and who not to spend time with without any guilt or remorse whatsoever. There are plenty of people willing to wallow in misery all of their lives, having endless conversations about what is wrong in the world, politics, the environment, their family, work, etc. It is more of a treasure to find someone willing to bring sunshine and strength wherever they go. Be that treasure! Be that sunshine. Be that strong positive anchor and never apologize for it! Just remember that being present and supportive when a person is temporarily going through a hard time is much different than buying into their negative world view.

If you choose to have a significant other, be mindful about your choice and be totally honest with yourself about why you want to be with this person. If you are not already in a relationship, ask yourself when you want this to happen? Do you feel you want to change some things in your life first? Do you feel you have to be perfectly healthy before you attract the right partner? Be realistic and throw away the idea that anyone has to be perfect. It is good to be on the journey to be the best person you can be but there is no need to wait until you have "arrived" at that place to have the partnership you may want.

Also, be aware that others are also on a journey. If you start to get to know someone and are attracted to them, notice where they are on their journey. Do they have a commitment to always learn and grow? Do they feel they have already accomplished all they want in life and are uninterested in developing any further? No matter where the two of you are right now, if only one of you has a commitment to personal growth and well-being, long term compatibility may be a challenge.

How do you feel when you are around your significant other? Do you stick around because you feel obligated, scared to be alone, or because you are truly a good match? What are some qualities that you want to be sure to have in a life partner or significant other? Take some time to write these things down.

Make sure when you write these things down that you are precise and know exactly what you mean. For example, if you write, "honest", what do you really mean? What about saying someone is dependable? What does that actually mean to you and what will you observe to determine whether you believe that person is dependable or not? Be very specific when you write down what you must have in a relationship. Next, write down how exactly you will know when you have this in positive terms (forms of "will not", "no", etc. are not allowed in the description). Only write down exactly what you want to see in simple terms. Next, write down things you prefer in a partner but is not a requirement. This may range from a hair color to being a vegan to speaking another language.

Now, let yourself be open to meeting this person anywhere. Become interested in people! Think about your closest connections right now. Where did you meet them?   Most likely it came naturally when you were going about your every day life. Make yourself available to more positive connections of all kinds. Make eye contact and really be open with others regardless of whether they are homeless or a celebrity. There is always something to learn from everybody. Observe people and ask questions. You never know when or where a new friend, love interest, or connection may be made.

Chapter 9

Savor the Taste Of Success

I fear not the man who has practiced 10,000 kicks once, but I fear the man who has practiced one kick 10,000 times. -Bruce Lee

The most important thing is to enjoy your life- to be happy- it's all that matters. - Audrey Hepburn

We must do the very best we can. This is our sacred responsibility. Most people tiptoe through life trying to safely make it to death.
-Albert Einstein

Do you realize what a huge difference changing just one habit for the rest of your life can do for your health, and life? One habit as simple as drinking pure water first thing in the morning, eating some healthy food within half an hour of waking in the morning, or always eating at least one fruit or vegetable with your evening meal can make a huge difference. It can increase how many years you live, make it so your body naturally maintains a lower weight, and give you energy to enjoy life.

Make sure this new healthy habit is something you are going to take action and do from now on and not something you are going to restrict! Whatever you do, make sure your new exercise or fitness routine is fun! It is much easier to stick to a new habit until it becomes a permanent lifestyle if it brings you joy!

Think of one fun activity that you would like to do more often. This is your chance to do all of the fun things you have wanted to give yourself permission to do! There are no limits- include any type of exercise that comes to mind- dancing, horseback riding, weight lifting, walking or running on the beach, hiking in the mountains, yoga, barre, pole dancing, swimming, and martial arts are just some examples of fun types of exercises to try.

When you exercise, do you enjoy exercising alone or exercising with others? Competing or being in a "zen" state? Exercising outside or indoors? Decide on one new, FUN activity that you will try every week until you find at least one that you love enough to do regularly. You deserve to do what you enjoy and become more healthy while you do it.

What do you love about yourself? **Your motivation to be healthy and fit is stronger and longer lasting when you are driven towards a goal you are excited about rather than doing something because you want to avoid feeling bad about yourself.**

Feeling healthy, having more energy, being able to play with your kids or play a sport, or living longer are some positively focused goals. It is good to move towards positive goals from a positive mindset. Take time today to notice and appreciate the good and the beauty in yourself and in every aspect of your life and your motivation will have so much more power and be long lasting!

Think about it. If you had everything you could ever imagine- a perfect relationship, the best friends in the world, all the money and security you want, accomplishment in whatever you set out to do, etc., yet were bedridden or feeling sickly for the rest of your life, what would matter most?

It is really hard to imagine having poor health when you are healthy unless you or someone close to you has gone through an illness and have come to the realization of how incredibly important it is to have a healthy body. It can literally be a matter of life and death!

When I was 37 years old, I became very sick for almost two months. I did everything possible to get better- went to the doctor, ate very healthfully, drank lots of alkaline water and vegetable juice, used natural remedies, rested as much as possible, breathed fresh air as much as possible, appreciated the positive & caring people around me, and let myself feel as positive and peaceful as possible. It still took me months to recover and be able to get out of bed just to take a short walk with deep breaths some days.

That experience really made me realize how pointless it was to over-stress myself in my life and ignore my health. In retrospect, I realized that I had been overly stressed from a very negative work environment that not only affected my mental health but had started affecting my physical health as well. It is a good reminder of how incredibly important my health is and how much energy and happiness and confidence that health brings.

Make small habit changes every week that you can keep on doing for the rest of your life. As you make these changes, make sure you are doing it primarily for yourself rather than from others reaction to your changes. Share your vibrant, healthy life more fully with your loved ones and have more energy to put into whatever your life purpose is- both personal, and professional! You are worth it! Take care of your health always! It is most likely the one thing you have most control over. Focus on what you want in life and for your body rather than what you don't want. Enjoy and treasure the good moments in life. Stop and smell every rose, and ignore the garbage. Get into the habit of doing it so often that all you notice are the beautiful roses in your life!

You have already proved your dedication by reading this book and beginning your journey. I hope you feel proud all that you have accomplished so far! Please think of it as just the beginning- you are integrating the basics of what it takes to develop and keep a healthy lifestyle deep inside yourself. Now there will be more challenges, you will have more decisions of your own to make. A major key to success is to never ever give up and to always promise yourself to learn and grow. Enjoy who you have become right now, and always have a goal as to what you want to do next. Above all, enjoy the process of learning and growing.

Think of a time in your life when you were in the process of accomplishing or learning something important. Look back and realize how precious those times were and love the younger you who was going through that process. **Realize that right NOW, you are going through a similar process and are a younger version of yourself working towards a better future. Your future self will look back and treasure these moments and thank you one day.** Stay humble and appreciate the peace that comes with knowing that good things are already in motion!

Just keep on putting one foot in front of the other NO MATTER WHAT and have fun with this process of following and living your dreams!

Chapter 10

Your Personalized Fitness Plan

You are about to create a one-day outline of what your ideal healthy day will look like. Sit down in the most comfortable and quiet place in your home, coffee shop, or even outside on a blanket. Make yourself some cool lemon water, hot herbal tea, or something else that will nourish your body and soul. Enjoy this process of exploring your ideal day from beginning to end. This will be your personalized fitness plan that you can enjoy using for the rest of your life!

By answering the following questions to the best of your ability, you will have created your own personalized fitness plan:

What will I focus my mind, heart, and soul on upon first waking up in the morning?
This may include a prayer, saying out loud what you are grateful for, creating your own mantra, and what you aim to be and experience during that day. Write this on your mirror, paper, or something that your eyes will see first thing in the morning.

What kind of physical activity will I do within half an hour of waking up in the morning?
This could be anything from a 2 minute stretch and showering, going on a brief walk outside, or going directly to the gym first thing in the morning.

How will I nourish my body upon waking each morning?
I recommend that you drink pure water when you first wake up. Something that has worked for me is drinking 8-10 ounces of water immediately upon waking (within 1-2 minutes). This flushes the system and wakes the body up. You could try adding fresh squeezed lemon or apple cider vinegar as well.

Nourish your body within 30 minutes of waking EACH MORNING. You may not feel hungry during the first few days of doing this. Do it anyway! It will help you be less hungry later in the day, when your body needs less calories. I once ran a weekly weight loss group for people whose goal was to lose 50 pounds or more. I ran this group for many cycles with many types of people. Ironically the number one thing everyone initially had in common regardless of their age, sex, and any other variable was that every single person either skipped breakfast or ate nothing until several hours after waking. There were different reasons- not hungry, feel like they would rather use the allotted calories for later in the day, etc. But everybody either skipped breakfast, ate breakfast more than 30 minutes after waking, and usually did not include protein and healthy foods in their breakfast. They changed this and started to see results. Make sure that you eat a breakfast with protein within 30 minutes of waking. Write down what you will drink and some options of what you may eat for breakfast daily.

What supplements (if any) will I take?

I recommend getting a blood test and physical and letting a primary care doctor advise you for supplements and assess for possible deficiencies (vitamin D, B12, calcium, etc.). If you already have done this and know your needs, please supplement your body accordingly. Make sure you take your supplements with food when recommended.

How will I manage stress throughout my day?
(both proactively and when unexpected stressful situations arise)

How will I fulfill my emotional and relational needs throughout the day?
(we have talked about this in other chapters)

What will I eat throughout the day for lunch, dinner, and snacks, and approximately when will I eat it?
You will likely need to play with this and re-adjust during the process of finding out what best nurtures your body. Feel free to write down how you will start out with this question and change it accordingly.

What emotional and mental state will I allow myself to be in when I eat?
(e.g. watching TV, anxious, busy, calm, centered, around people who I tend to feel nervous around, around people who eat when they are in a fully present state of being, etc.)

What kind of foods can I eat that are both delicious to me and healthy?

How and when will I prepare my meals?
Will you prepare your meals at home every day? What types of meals will you prepare? Will you make healthy lunches for you and your family on the weekend and freeze them so that they are ready to go? When would you like to get groceries? What restaurants might you go to and what delicious and healthy things might you order when you do go out?

Do I want to offer a prayer, blessing, or center myself before eating a meal?
This not only connects you spiritually, it can also ground and center you, which can protect from overeating depending on your personal triggers.

How much sleep do I need to feel energized every day and how will I get the sleep that my body needs?

How much water will I drink and approximately what times during the day will I drink the water?
Making sure your body is hydrated does wonders to your energy levels, health, and can sometimes reduce cravings. Notice your body. Do you start to crave sweets when you are dehydrated? If you start to feel sleepy in the middle of the day, does drinking water help? It is best not to drink large amounts of water (especially ice water) during meals because it slows digestion and absorption of nutrients. I suggest drinking water throughout the day.

How will I prevent or prepare for cravings by eating healthy snacks or meals while cravings are still manageable?

What types of activity will I engage in throughout the day?
What, when, and where will I do cardio, stretching, and/or weight training? Will you take a break from your desk every hour? Sit on a ball or do pushups in the middle of the day to boost your energy?

What types of individual needs does my body have that would be good to pay special attention to?
For example, do you have any injuries or illnesses that require special care? Do you have a tendency towards a deficiency? Do you require more rest, more quiet time, or more movement than the average person? Do you need chiropractic care, acupuncture, physical therapy, or other alternative therapies?

Do I tend to get cold or hot easily? If so, how do I keep my body regulated? Do I need a special chair or back support while working at a desk or driving?

When have I been most likely to binge in the past? What prompts this?
Take your time with this question and write down how you are feeling emotionally, physically, spiritually, mentally before binges in the past. Do you feel like something is missing in your life? How do you feel about yourself right before you have binged? Once you know these things, you can address and resolve these things in a fulfilling and healthy way before the desire to binge occurs.

Are my mental and emotional needs being taken care of?
Am I overworked and analytical when my brain would benefit from relaxation and creativity more in my life? Do I need to start incorporating more excitement, more connection, or more of anything else in my life?

Am I feeling fulfilled spiritually?
If not, what can do I do in order to change this?

Am I feeling fulfilled sexually?
If not, what can I do in order to change this?

Am I feeling fulfilled in my relationships with others and myself?
If not, what can I do in order to change this?

What would make me feel even more happy and fulfilled in my life?

Do I have love, peace, and joy as my primary emotions throughout my day?
If not, what can I do in order to change this?

When am I most likely to need a boost of love, peace, and joy?
Make a flexible schedule of how you will take care of all your needs throughout the day.

Feel free to add more of your own questions in order to outline things that you would like to incorporate into your ideal healthy day.

Now, incorporate the things you have recorded above during the next full day and record how you feel and how things work out throughout this test day.

Did drinking water first thing in the morning and throughout the day seem to give you a big unexpected boost of energy? Did you find exercising in the morning is not for you and you would rather release stress during the day or at a yoga class directly after work instead? Experiment with what works best for you.

The main skill to learn is to listen carefully to your body and become an expert in anticipating what you really need before it becomes so strong so that you take care of yourself in an unhealthy way. Avoid restricting or starving yourself. Take care of yourself and treasure yourself. This will lead to amazing feelings of health that will radiate throughout your entire being for the rest of your life!

SHRINK WORKBOOK

Become Bulletproof. Move Mountains.

Create a Revolution Inside Your Body For The World To See!

Every week, work on one assignment. Repeat or work on the assignment or activity every day during the entire week.

Week 1: Meet the New You!

Remember that you create and shape exactly who you are. Your thoughts, emotions, and decisions every second of every day are extremely powerful and little by little have created the body and lifestyle that keep your body the way it is. The very first step is to imagine what you really want your body to look like and feel like.

Take at least 15 completely undisturbed minutes every day this week in a place that makes you feel peaceful. It could be a park, the sandy beach, a grassy yard, your sunny front porch, or your most comfortable couch (as long as the TV is off and no other people will be visible or make any distracting noises). Make sure you are away from all distracting sounds, smells, and sights. Sit comfortably and breath in and out through your mouth with your mouth open throughout this exercise.

Visualize in detail your ideal self living in your ideal body two years from now. You have created this gorgeous, beautiful body that expresses your ideal self who has always been who you really are deep down. Take all the time you want to enjoy these feelings of walking, moving, talking, exercising, riding in the car, eating, sleeping and doing other everyday activities in your new, healthy body. Savor every movement and sink into this new feeling of moving freely and being joyful with how your body moves as you walk, sit, or play. Enjoy the satisfying and peaceful feeling of breathing in fresh air deeply into your lungs.   Just think about this vividly and bask in these blissful feelings for about 10 minutes or whenever you feel ready for the next exercise.

Now, imagine looking at yourself in the mirror as you move and enjoy the new, happy, physically fit person you see. Notice your reflection in detail.

Notice the colors, the shapes, your body language and facial expression. Maybe you notice yourself in a window reflection as you are walking. Let yourself feel deeply happy, peaceful, and grounded about your body and the lifestyle you have created as you see your reflection. Think about all of the things you have accomplished in your life as a result of having energy, radiant health, and confidence. Notice how much you have been able to contribute to the world with your renewed energy, confidence, and health!

Take a good look at the powerful, energetic, and attractive body you have created through your thoughts, feelings, habits. Let yourself feel good about having created your healthy body. Soak in all of those good feelings about yourself. Let go of anything else that comes up. In this exercise, only focus on the delicious, satisfying feelings that come up when looking at your reflection.

Now, close your eyes and just let the thoughts, sounds, feelings, and sight of your new body and lifestyle sink in. Spend some time now deeply and throughly enjoying these feelings and emotions!

Week 2:
What Gives you Super Human Strength?

On day 1 of this week, write down one sentence saying what your main health-related goal is for the week. Make it simple and measurable. Make the sentence so easy to understand that a first grader could both read it and know when it has been met.

Every day of this week, write down a paragraph or two about WHY you made this change in your life and how your life has changed now. Really get into it and enjoy explaining how this made you accomplish your lifelong goal. Make sure to write down why you changed as though you have already done this (past tense). Make sure to do this every day.

Now every day this week, take a short ten minute walk and think about how good your body feels after having made this change you wrote about. Make the effort to keep smiling for the entire ten minute walk! This is more challenging than you may think. Make sure you put forth the effort to keep a smile on your face and bask in the good feelings you get when intensely imagining your new body and lifestyle during this 10 minute walk. As silly as this may sound, actually writing this out and taking this smiling walk does wonders internally.

Week 3: Get acquainted with yourself

Every day this week, go through this list of
questions for 30-60 minutes. Get to know
yourself while giving yourself unconditional love.
There are no right or wrong answers. Only
discovery and progress. Enjoy the journey of
understanding yourself better!

• What are your earliest food memories?
• What were your family's eating and exercising
  patterns?

• How was food used in your family?

• When you became old enough to buy and
  prepare your own food, what did you buy and
  prepare?

• What messages did you hear about food and
  weight growing up?

• What did you expect to feel or become from
  what you ate?

• What things can I do immediately to reduce my
  stress?

- Which mindsets will help me reduce and manage my stress?
- What is my life purpose?

- Am I living a life that keeps my purpose at the core?

- What do I value the most in life?

- How do I keep my values in mind when making decisions?

- Do I feel that my values and actions are in agreement? If not, this is likely producing great amounts of stress (cognitive dissonance).

- What things can I do to begin to turn around and eliminate the big stressors in my life (for example if your personality isn't a good fit for customer service, starting process of changing careers, etc.)? Although a drastic change in a given area may not always be able to be made tomorrow, a decision regarding what is acceptable/how to deal with situations, and steps towards that decision can be made immediately (e.g. steps for preparing for qualification for a new job, speaking to a coworker or spouse about something that stresses you out, etc.).

- What are the pros and cons (cost/benefit) of reducing the biggest things that produce stress for me?

- What is my highest goal in life?

- Do I have other goals, values, or obligations that seem to go against meeting this goal? If so, how will I go about resolving it? What do they both have in common?

- Do I hold onto stress because I feel it motivates me?

- How can I get the same result of feeling motivated in a more positive way?

- How can I focus on my desire/goal so intensely so that I am magnetically drawn to do everything within my power to meet this goal?

- How can I organize my life so that my exercise, rest, healthy relationships that I've developed, and my nutrition actually reduces my stress rather than adds to it (this can be done with the help of an expert in nutrition, exercise, psychology, etc.)?

Week 4: How to Become the Expert

Every day this week, schedule two times during each day that you routinely "check in" with yourself. What times of day do you usually feel most like overeating? Set the alarm on your phone for those two times each day when you are most likely to feel like overeating. It doesn't have to be exact, just pick a time.

When your alarm rings each day, read the following 15 questions and answer them silently. Get into the habit of noticing your body, mind, and spirit and what you need. Immediately fulfill and take care of the underlying desires and cravings as much as possible.

Get into the habit of doing this every day even after you move on to next week's assignment.

1. Do I have tension anywhere in my body right now? If so, what is it telling me? What do I need to do to relieve that tension?

2. Am I worrying or longing for something?

3. Am I feeling lonely, sad, angry, or overwhelmed? If so, what can I do or give myself to feel better?

4. If I could have anything besides food right now, what would it be? How can I give this to myself?

5. Could my body use some water right now (ask this especially if you are craving sweets)?

6. Do I need sleep or relaxation?

7. Would it feel good for me to take some deep breaths of fresh air?

8. Would it feel good to move around, stretch, exercise, or change positions?

9. Do I crave companionship or connection with someone?

10. What would I like to emotionally share with somebody?

11. Am I feeling bored? What exciting thing would I rather be doing?

12. What would make me feel most treasured or valued right now?

13. Do I feel good about what I am accomplishing today?

14. Do I feel recognized and respected for who I am?

15. What other cravings or needs are coming up for me right now?

Week 5: Your Gold Medal

Write down one concrete goal to accomplish by the end of this week. Make sure it is an action you will do (not of a measurement or appearance of your body). This is an assignment for starting a new action and making it permanent, not for restricting yourself. These two things work differently in your mind so be attentive to what new healthy habit you are beginning and always focus on positive actions you are taking.

For example, you could use a goal of completing two yoga or Zumba classes, working up to hiking your favorite trail, playing tag outside with your child for 30 minutes by the end of the week, walking for 45 minutes on the beach without stopping, eating 5 servings of vegetables every day, allowing for 8 hours of sleep each night, drinking a certain amount of water each day, or completing a 5k. Make it something you used to enjoy or something you have always wanted to try or be able to do. Write it down below and formulate your own plan of action to make this happen by the end of the week. Make sure it is a goal that you are able to prepare for and accomplish within one week.

Week 6: Try some samples and experiment!

Take 10 minutes on day 1 to write down 20-100 health-related things you have never done before that you are willing to try! Your assignment for the rest of this week is to try as many new things on this list as possible. Try so many that you "fail" and find out what you do not enjoy. You have not completed this assignment until you have tried at least 10 new health-related things that you are not interested in doing regularly.

For example, you may sample essential oils, attending a weight loss support group, juicing, a yoga class, a vegan cooking class, a new fruit or vegetable you have not eaten before, a new sport such as fencing, swimming, hiking, a deep tissue massage, using a sea salt scrub in the shower, trying out different veggie smoothies or healthy recipes, water aerobics, pole dancing, or dodgeball. Try everything you can think of that would remotely interest you at least once!

You can find hundreds of things to do that are free! When making the list, try out new things that might be best for you in your life right now. You will probably find some new interests or habits that you like and start doing it regularly.

Only YOU can find what is perfect for YOUR body, mind, and spirit.

Make sure you notice and write about how your body feels (chest, stomach, head, etc.), as well as what emotions and thoughts come up for you as you try each new thing.

For example, if you have never lifted weights before, schedule a session with a personal trainer or friend and lift weights for the first time. If you have never been to a yoga class, go to a beginner yoga class. Some examples of how you may feel during these experiences may include cold, warm, centered, uncoordinated, balanced, strong, beautiful, capable, etc. You may feel some emotions in the pit of your stomach, your upper chest, muscles in your neck and shoulders, etc. The possibilities are endless. The point is to pay attention to how your body reacts and listen to your body's experience after doing something you wouldn't have ordinarily done. This is how you experiment and find out what you love and what is best for you.

Week 7: Reframe to become invincible!

Each day this week, write down at least one thing you can think of that you "failed" at in the course of your life.

Now beside each "failure", write down at least one thing you have learned from each "failure" that actually makes you more wise and/or powerful today. Reframe these "failures" in your mind into circumstances that were a blessing in disguise that taught you life's great lessons to make you better and improve your game. Recognize how these "failures" may prevent you from making future mistakes.

Week 7 Daily Journaling Exercise:

Day	"Failure"	How it makes me wiser
1.		
2.		
3.		
4.		
5.		
6.		
7.		

Week 8: What are your three wishes?

You find a genie who promises to give you three wishes in your life. Write a few paragraphs about what these three things are and how having these things in your life could fulfill your deepest craving. Pay close attention to what feelings you anticipate these things will bring you. These feelings are the keys to what your soul's deepest cravings are. Take full ownership of what you truly want in your life, giving yourself love and unconditional acceptance as your soul's deepest cravings come up. Make a picture in your mind of receiving these things. Make it big, colorful, and beautiful like an IMAX movie. Make it so vivid that you are almost experiencing it right now. Welcome these things into your life!

Now, think and reflect on of how being at a healthy body weight and being physically fit will or won't change your life. What will having a fit and healthier body do or not do for you? Take a few undisturbed moments to go outside and sit under a shady tree or in the sunshine. Close your eyes and think about what you imagine your life to be like 2-3 months from now, when you are well on your way to living the healthy life you have imagined and created. Write down the highlights. Also, write down what it prompts you to do differently or change today if anything. What are you aware of now that you weren't aware of before? What parts of yourself are you more aware of? What would you like to express or share with others? What would you like to develop more of within yourself?

Week 9: Who are your biggest cheerleaders?

Surround yourself with those who support, challenge, and motivate you.

Write Down the names of the 2-5 closest people to you who you believe will be truly and unconditionally supportive of you as you create your new lifestyle. If you do not have at least 2 people like this in your life right now, congratulations on recognizing this and being truthful. Starting from scratch may be a blessing in disguise!

Top 5 people who are unconditionally supportive to me:

1.

2.

3.

4.

5.

Now, write down a list of 10 qualities you want to see in someone in order to consider them a truly supportive, trustworthy, and dependable part of your "entourage" during this transition in your life.

Top Qualities I want to see in my inner circle:

1.

2.

3.

4.

5.

6.

7.

8.

9.

10.

Week 10. Celebrate your success!

Every day this week, recognize at least one positive thing you have done to improve your health for that day. Celebrating success anchors it into your life.

Now celebrate this success and spend the rest of the day celebrating and feeling deep gratitude for having done this!

How did you celebrate your successes?

Congratulations for being on the path to success! You have successfully gone through the process of creating a revolution inside your body for the world to see! This process is a great adventure. It is journey, so re-read sections when you feel you need a boost or refresher. And remember that health is a lifestyle process, not a destination. Enjoy your magnificent body at every stage of this journey.

Please continue paying attention to big and small successes. Celebrating them as soon as you recognize it both with immense energy, smiles, and letting yourself experience immediate joy! Pay attention to your heart and mind and focus on what you can be grateful for each day.

Stay connected to this Inside Out Fitness community and receive more resources and support at insideoutfitness.com. Enjoy the process of becoming bulletproof, dropping the deadweight in your life, and thriving in your new personalized way of life. From the bottom of my heart, I wish you a happy, healthy, and long life.

Warmly,

Dr. Daphne

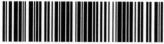

Made in the USA
San Bernardino, CA
28 May 2018